CLASSIC
RADIOLOGIC
SIGNS

CLASSIC RADIOLOGIC SIGNS

An atlas and history

MICHAEL E. MULLIGAN

Assistant Professor, Diagnostic Radiology,
University of Maryland, School of Medicine

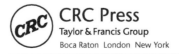

CRC Press
Taylor & Francis Group
Boca Raton London New York

CRC Press is an imprint of the
Taylor & Francis Group, an **informa** business

CRC Press
Taylor & Francis Group
6000 Broken Sound Parkway NW, Suite 300
Boca Raton, FL 33487-2742

First issued in paperback 2019

© 1997 by Taylor & Francis Group, LLC
CRC Press is an imprint of Taylor & Francis Group, an Informa business

No claim to original U.S. Government works

ISBN-13: 978-1-85070-664-9 (hbk)
ISBN-13: 978-0-367-40115-3 (pbk)

Visit the Taylor & Francis Web site at
http://www.taylorandfrancis.com

and the CRC Press Web site at
http://www.crcpress.com

DEDICATION

This book is dedicated to
all radiologists and
their fanciful imaginations,
especially to Wilhelm Conrad Röntgen
who made it all possible

TABLE OF CONTENTS

PREFACE

Radiology is a visual art. Since the discovery of the X-ray in 1895, many of the radiographic patterns we see have been given catchy descriptive names that are supposed to help us remember and recognize certain disease patterns or entities. A few textbooks have been written that catalog more than 400 of these terms. In honor of the 100th anniversary of Röntgen's discovery of the X-ray, this book will illustrate and elaborate on the history of 100 of the more classic (or soon to be classic) radiologic signs. If we are to be able to use these terms with full understanding, we must visualize the object depicted by the term, imagine its radiographic appearance and transfer that picture to the radiographic image before us. This book is intended to help all students and practitioners of our art accomplish that task.

The following sentiments, expressed by Mark Ravitch[1], regarding eponyms apply equally well to many of the terms to be described in this book:

> My own feeling is that whatever their fallibility, eponyms illuminate the lineage of surgery and bring to it the color of old times, distinguished figures, ancient sieges, and pestilences, and continually remind us of the international nature of science.

> Fallible eponyms certainly may be. Given an eponym one may be sure (1) that the man so honored was not the first to describe the disease, the operation, or the instrument, or (2) that he misunderstood the situation, or (3) that he is generally misquoted, or (4) that (1), (2), and (3) are all simultaneously true ...

> Priority, in the award of an eponym, is not necessarily purely temporal: ... in terms

of importance to medicine and to the sick, the physician who convinces his colleagues of the value of a new procedure, which they then adopt, exceeds in significance his hapless fellow who devised the same procedure earlier but failed to gain its adoption. And by the same token, the individual who first clearly establishes the nature of a condition is usually more deserving of the eponym than the forgotten author of a mere description unearthed by diligent scholasticism or pure serendipity.

With diligent scholasticism and some serendipity, I have carefully tried to track down the first use or first appearance in print of these terms or their antecedents. The original articles and books were used whenever they were available to me. There is no doubt that some terms were in use long before their 'documentation' in the literature. Any errors or misappropriations are my own and I accept full responsibility for them. I did not try to document the first description of each disease entity. That would have doubled my chances of being wrong. Other books dealing with the history of medicine have compiled that type of information. For those of you who would quarrel with my assertions about who reported what, please keep in mind the maxims of Mark Ravitch[1] quoted above.

Many of the terms described in this book have been used for more than one abnormality over the last 100 years. I have described in detail only one usage of the term that I considered most appropriate for this book. Some people will not agree that the terms I have selected are the most classic. Others will be disappointed when they do not find their favorite sign in the book. In reply, I would say that the choices were sometimes difficult. The origins of several classic terms (eg. cannon-ball metastases, butterfly glioma, stepladder bowel loops and drooping lily), I could not discover. This fact will account for some omissions. Perhaps the 200th anniversary edition will contain all the other classics of yesterday and tomorrow.

Reference
1. Ravitch, M.M. (1979). Dupuytren's invention of the Mikulicz enterotome with a note on eponyms. *Perspect. Biol. Med.*, 22, 170–84

ACKNOWLEDGEMENTS

Many people have helped to make this book possible. Past and present colleagues, especially those at the University of Maryland and the Armed Forces Institute of Pathology (AFIP), reviewed my proposed lists of classic signs to help ensure that they were indeed among the classics. The final choices were my own, however, I would especially like to thank Anne Brower, Jim Buck, Erik Cameron, Melissa Christenson-Rosado, Abe Dachmann, Doug Fellows, Dave Hartmann, Barbara Miller, Mark Murphey, Charles Resnik, Jim Smirniotopolous, Phil Templeton and Charles White for their suggestions. Lent Johnson deserves special mention for background information on bone-tumor terms that he provided. Many of the terms described in this book have been used for more than one abnormality, I have described in detail the usage that I considered most appropriate.

Acquiring the background materials and original articles or texts was a monumental task. I must thank Sue Mosteller for her numerous trips to the Health Sciences Library (HSL) at the University of Maryland where she retrieved and copied many of the articles for this book. The librarians at many other institutions were also most helpful. The resources available to me at the HSL, National Library of Medicine (NLM), Johns Hopkins Welch Medical Library and non-medical libraries in the University of Maryland System were invaluable and if they didn't have a particular article, the interlibrary loan system made it available. Steve Greenberg in the History Division of the NLM is a most knowledgeable, capable and helpful fellow. Nancy Knight and Vickie Giannotti at the American College of Radiology (ACR) Center for the History of Radiology provided access to some key materials.

Many of the original articles were in foreign language journals, most notably German, French, Spanish and Italian. Since my own language background included only Latin and Spanish, I had to rely on professional translators both human and computer based to extract much of the important information. Ms Frances Kleeman provided excellent translations of several German and French articles, so too did the Power Translator Professional computer programs of Globalink Inc. Drs Maria Pace, Jose Novoa and Barbara Jaeger also helped tremendously, as did Rose Jaeger and Petra Flick. My thanks also go to Drs Luis F. Mattoso and Juan Chifflet for their help in reference sourcing. Dr Robert Allman reviewed the original draft of the manuscript and had many helpful suggestions for improving it.

A radiology book without pictures is as useful as a television without a picture tube. Mr David Crandall took or reproduced more than half of the photos used to illustrate this work, as the list of photograph credits indicates. We are most fortunate to have him within our Department of Radiology at the University of Maryland.

My thanks to the various journal and book publishers, authors and corporations for permission to use the original photographs, illustrations and logos needed to illustrate this book.

Ms Linda Clarke typed the manuscript and numerous revisions promptly and expertly.

My thanks to Mr Charley Mitchell for his help in finding a publisher, and to the people at the Parthenon Publishing Group for undertaking this task.

Finally, my deepest gratitude to my wife and son for their love, patience and understanding over the many months it took to complete this book.

APPLE CORE (NAPKIN RING) LESION

Several different terms have been used to describe annular carcinomas of the colon. Raoul Bensaude and Georges Guénaux[1] in 1916 said 'a typical finding with cancer is when the shadow [of contrast] narrows to a small bridge between two broad shadows, looking as if a chunk had been gouged out on each side.' The finding is recognized and reported as *typical* even though the 'first opaque enema as a method for X-ray examination of the colon'[2] had only been reported in 1904 by Schule[3]. One of the early masters of the bismuth enema (barium was introduced in 1910[4]) was Feodor Haenisch of Hamburg, Germany. He wrote about the early diagnosis of cancer of the colon and visited the US to teach his fluoroscopic technique. He described finger-like projections and thin streams of bismuth extending through the narrowed areas of carcinoma.[5,6] Russell Carman in a 1923 review of the roentgenologic signs of colon cancer, in 359 cases examined at the Mayo Clinic, used the term napkin ring in both the pathologic discussion and radiographic figure legends. He described this as a well-known form of scirrhus cancer (Figure 1). He emphasized that, 'Roentgenologic manifestations of cancer of the colon, as elicited by the opaque enema, are few and simple. Practically there are but two of importance, namely the filling defect and obstruction.' Apple core lesion (Figure 2) seems to be the preferred term at the viewbox today. (Napkin rings have disappeared from most of the dinner tables in our fast food society.)

The apple was known to the prehistoric inhabitants of Europe. Carbonized fruits have been found in the debris of Swiss and Italian lake dwellings. The original home of the apple *(Malus sylvestris)* is thought to be in the region south of the Caucasus. Apples were familiar to the Greeks and Romans, being mentioned by Theophrastus in the third century BC with the name 'Mailea' or 'Malus'. Variety lists of apples were available as early as 100 BC[8].

References
1. Bensaude, R. and Guénaux, G. (1916). Le radio-diagnostic du cancer du gros intestin. Cancer sans signes d'occlusion. *Arch. Mal. Appar. Digest. Mal. Nutr.*, 9, 179–220. Abstracted translation, *J. Am. Med. Assoc.*, 1917, 69, 155–6

2. Eisenberg, R.L. (1992). *Radiology – An Illustrated History*, p. 278. (St Louis: Mosby-Year Book Inc.)

3. Schule, A. (1904). Intubation and radiography of the large intestine. *Arch. Verdauungskr. Stoffwechselpathol. Diat*, 10, 111–18

4. Bachem, C. and Gunther, H. (1910). Barium sulfate as a shadow-forming contrast agent in roentgenologic examinations. *Z. Röntgenkd. Radiumforsch.*, 12, 369–76

5. Haenisch, G.F. (1911). Roentgenologic examination in narrowing of the large intestine: the early roentgenologic diagnosis of carcinoma of the large intestine. *Muenchen Med. Wschr.*, 45, 2331–75

6. Haenisch, F. (1911). The value of the roentgen ray in the early diagnosis of carcinoma of the bowel. *Am. Q. Roentgenol.*, 3, 175–80

7. Carman, R.D. (1923). Roentgenologic signs of cancer of the colon. *J. Radiol.*, 4, 147–51

8. Smock, R.M. and Neubert, A.M. (1950). *Apples and Apple Products.* (New York: Interscience Pub. Inc.)

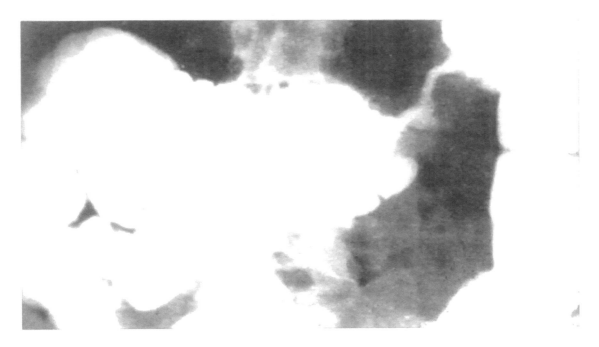

Figure 1. 'Napkin ring cancer of the transverse colon.' Reprinted from Carman'. Roentgenologic signs of cancer of the colon. *J. Radiology,* **4,** 147–51, with permission of the RSNA

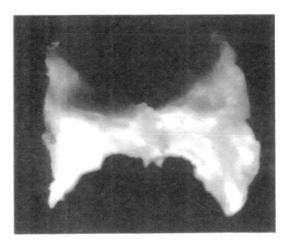

Figure 2. An apple core

ASTERISK SIGN

The quest for an early radiologic imaging sign of avascular necrosis continued despite Alex Norman's and Peter Bullough's 1963 report[1] of the crescent sign on plain radiographs and the development of radioisotope bone scanning (see Crescent sign). Wolfgang Dihlmann's contribution[2] to the quest was the description of an early computerized tomography (CT) sign – the asterisk sign – in 1982. He studied 71 patients and four gross specimens at the Institute of Roentgenology in Hamburg. He showed that the normal arrangement of the trabeculae in the femoral head was in the form of a small star or asterisk (Figure 1). 'The image of the asterisk of the femoral head in CT is formed by physiologically thickened load-transmitting bone trabeculae.'[2] The appearance of this asterisk was altered in patients with avascular necrosis before they had any changes evident on plain radiographs (Figure 2). 'The reduced mechanical loadability of dead bone trabeculae ... leads to (micro-) fractures which disturb the arrangement of the trabeculae and alter the form of the asterisk.'[2] This CT sign is useful, however, magnetic resonance imaging (MRI) has supplanted CT scanning for the early diagnosis of avascular necrosis and this sign is not used during MRI interpretation. MRI allows direct visualization of the changes within the marrow and does not rely on changes in trabecular structure.

Definitions of the word asterisk include, 'a little star' and 'the figure of a star (*) used in writing and printing.'[3] (Figure 3).

References

1. Norman, A. and Bullough P. (1963). The radiolucent crescent line – an early diagnostic sign of avascular necrosis of the femoral head. *Bull. Hosp. Joint Dis.*, 24, 99–104

2. Dihlmann, W. (1982). CT analysis of the upper end of the femur: the asterisk sign and ischaemic bone necrosis of the femoral head. *Skeletal Radiol.*, 8, 251–8

3. Simpson, J. and Weiner, E. (eds.) *Oxford English Dictionary*, 1989, 2nd edn., Vol. 1, p. 727. (Oxford: Clarendon Press)

Figure 1. Normal 'asterisk' pattern in femoral head. Reprinted from Dihlmann[2]. CT analysis of the upper end of the femur. *Skeletal Radiol.*, **8**, 251–8, with permission of Springer Verlag

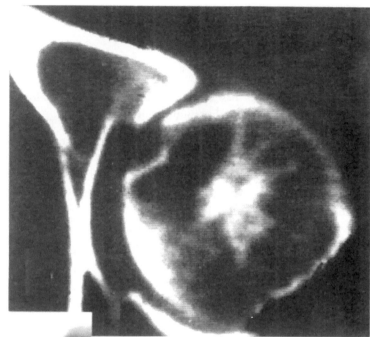

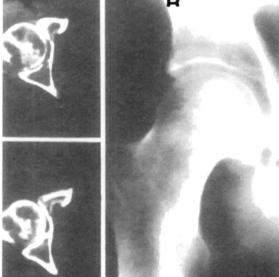

Figure 2. Early stage of avascular necrosis. 'Hyperdense spots and hyperdense streets running from the centre of the asterisk to the cortical bone, indicate the presence of [avascular necrosis]. The diagnosis ... was first established by CT' in this case. Reprinted from Dihlmann[2]. CT analysis of the upper end of the femur. *Skeletal Radiol.*, 1982, **8**, 251–8, with permission of Springer-Verlag

Figure 3. The printer's asterisk

BAMBOO SPINE

Ankylosing spondylitis has been recognized in skeletons found throughout the centuries. Bernard Connor (1666–1698), an Irishman, 'while demonstrating anatomy in France ... came across a most unusual skeleton found in a graveyard in which the ilium and sacrum and the 15 lowest vertebrae and adjoining ribs formed one continuous bone ... Connor fully realised the importance of his discovery and reported it in three languages, in French ... in Latin ... and in English ... By the late 1800s sufficient interest [allowed] Strümpell in 1884 to venture a tentative textbook mention, citing two patients with complete ankylosis of the spine and hip joints ... this was followed by ... papers by Strümpell (1897), von Bechterew (1893 and 1899) and Pierre Marie (1898).'[1]

Valentini is credited, by some, with the first radiographic description of the bamboo spine[2]. His 1899 article[3], 'Contribution on chronic, ankylosing inflammation of the spine and the hip joints', discusses the clinical and radiographic findings in five young men. The vertebral bodies were not distinguishable from each other. Shadows extended along both sides of the spinal column that blended the vertebral bodies with the ribs. The longitudinal ligaments were also thought to be calcified or ossified. Valentini acknowledged that the clinical observations of Pierre Marie[4] and Ernst Strümpell[5] preceded his own. Valentini did not use the term bamboo spine in his report. Dr Charles Buckley[6] credits Krebs as the originator of the bamboo-like analogy. Krebs, in his 1930 article[7], describes the radiographic appearance of the ankylosed spine as looking like a bamboo reed (bambusrohraussehen). Krebs pointed out many of the radiologic differences between ankylosing spondylitis and spondylitis deformans. This sign is pathogno-monic for ankylosing spondylitis (Figure 1).

This roentgen and pathologic classic sign likens the fused spinal segments with their syndesmophytes to a culm (stalk) of bamboo (Figure 2). *Bambusa ventricosa* (Figure 3) most closely resembles the fused spine of a patient with ankylosing spondylitis in this author's opinion. Bamboo refers to any of the tall tree-like grasses comprising the subfamily Bambusoideae of the family Poaceae. *B. ventricosa* is a shrub-like bamboo, native to China, with normal culms 2.5–5 m tall, 1–5.5 cm in diameter[8].

References
1. Moll, J.M.H. (1980). *Ankylosing Spondylitis*, pp. 2–6. (Edinburgh: Churchill Livingstone)
2. Berens, D.L. (1971). Roentgen features of ankylosing spondylitis. *Clin. Orthop.*, 74, 20–33
3. Valentini (1899). Beitrag zur chronischen, ankylosirenden Entzündung der Wirbelsäule und der Hüftgelenke. *Dtsch. Z. Nervenheilkd.*, 15, 239–49
4. Marie, P. (1898). Deux cas de spondylose rhizomélique. *Bull. Mem. Soc. Med. Hosp. Paris*, 15, 121–5
5. Strümpell, E.A. (1897). Bemerkung über die chronische ankylosirende Entzündung der Wirbelsäule und der Huftgelenke. *Dtsch. Z. Nervenheilkd.*, 11, 338–42
6. Buckley, C.W. (1931). Spondylitis deformans. *Br. Med. J.*, i, 1108–12
7. Krebs V. (1930). Zur Frage der Sogenannten rheumatischen Erknankungen der Wirbelsaüle. *Dtsch. Med. Wochenschr.*, 56, 220–22
8. Dajun, W. and Shao-Jin, S. (1987). *Bamboos of China*, p. 16. (Portland:Timber Press)

Figure 1. Anteroposterior radiograph showing ankylosis of vertebral segments resulting in bamboo spine appearance (author's case)

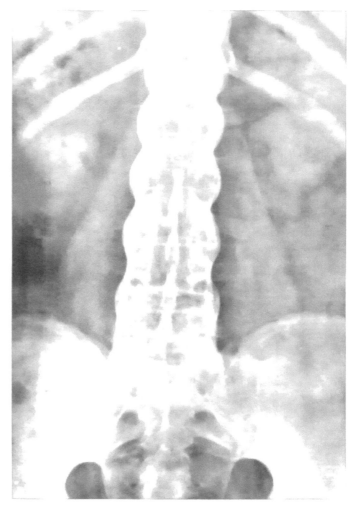

Figure 2. Bamboo stalks with nodes clearly visible

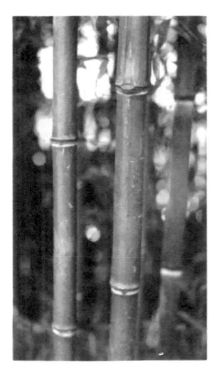

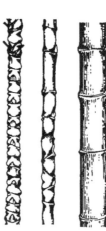

Figure 3. *Bambusa ventricosa, Phyllostachys aurea* and *Phyllostachys pubescens* (left to right) showing nodes and internodes, forms, sizes and lengths in proportion. Reprinted with permission from *Bamboos of China* by Dajun and Shao-Jin (1987)[8]. Copyright 1987 by Timber Press. All rights reserved

BEAK (CLAW) SIGN

It is obvious that renal lumps or bumps may not always be dromedary humps (see Dromedary kidney). The differentiation of a renal-cyst hump from a renal-neoplasm lump is important but not always easy even with the use of newer techniques like ultrasound, computerized tomography and magnetic resonance imaging.

Jacques Dautrebande and colleagues[1] (Montreal) credit ' Olle Olsson[2] (University Hospital, Lunde, Sweden) for describing one differentiator, the beak or claw sign. This was originally an angiographic sign (Figure 1). In the 1950s–1960s, angiograms were frequently performed, once a renal mass was discovered, to further delineate its nature. The term can now be used during the nephrogram phase of high quality excretory urography (usually on nephrotomograms) when a mass is seen. The findings are the same as those Olsson described on angiograms; 'The most important characteristics of a cyst are seen in the nephrographic phase ... A typical feature is the spur formation seen in the margin of the filling defect. This is formed by the renal parenchyma bordering the cyst and is due to displacement by the growing non infiltrative cyst. This raised margin ... is seen as a spur or beak in tangential projections ... if the angiogram [nephrogram] shows a well-defined avascular region with a beak-shaped border to the parenchyma, the lesion is a cyst.'[2]

Nephrotomography was introduced by John Evans and co-workers[3] in 1954. Although von Lichtenberg and Swick[4] reported the use of intravenous urography in 1929, 'a practical intravenous technique for obtaining a nephrogram was not evolved until 1951, when it was described by Weens, et al.'[5]

'The earliest known bird was Archaeopteryx. Five almost complete fossils of this ancient bird have been found in late Jurassic limestone about 150 million years old.'[6] Since Archaeopteryx was part reptile and part bird, there were teeth in its jaw as well as feathers on its wings. Modern birds' beaks are toothless but specialized and quite varied from species to species (Figure 2).

The term, beak sign, has also been used to describe the appearance of the distal esophagus in patients with achalasia.

References
1. Dautrebande, J., Duckett, G. and Roy, P. (1967). The claw sign of cortical cysts in renal arteriography. *J. Can. Assoc. Radiol.*, 18, 240–50

2. Olsson, O. (1961). Renal tumor and cyst. In Abrams, H.L. (ed.) *Angiography*, pp. 557–68. (Boston: Little Brown and Co.)

3. Evans, J.A., Dubilier, W. and Monteith, J.C. (1954). Nephrotomography: a preliminary report. *Am. J. Roentgenol.*, 71, 213–23

4. von Lichtenberg, A. and Swick, M. (1929). Klinische prüfung des Uroselectans. *Klin. Wchnschr.*, 8, 2089–91. Cited by Bertin, E.J. (1946). In Unusual urinary calculi. *Am. J. Roentgenol.*, 55, 181–8

5. Pfister, R.C. and Shea, T.E. (1971). Nephrotomography. *Radiol. Clin. North Am.*, 9, 41–62

6. King, A.S. and McLelland, J. (1984). *Birds – Their Structure and Function*, p.1. (London: Baillière Tindall)

7. Abrams, H. L. (1961). *Angiography*. (Boston: Little Brown and Co.)

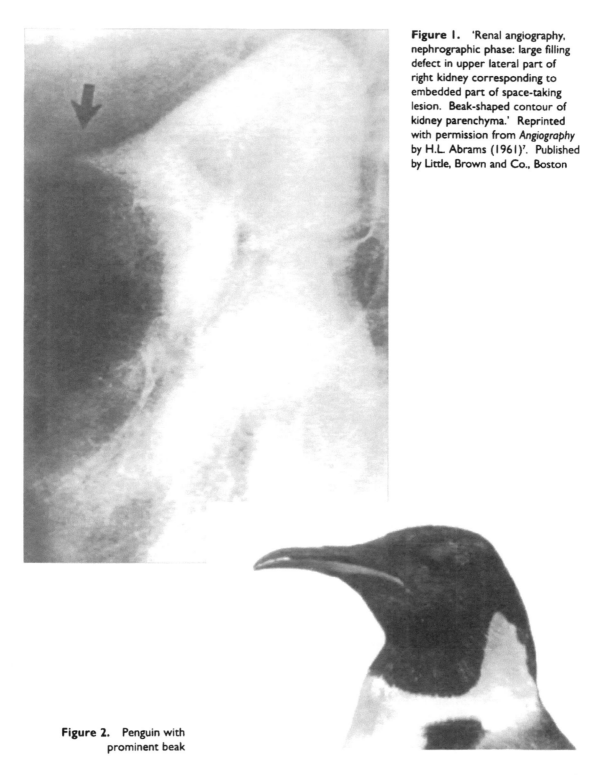

Figure 1. 'Renal angiography, nephrographic phase: large filling defect in upper lateral part of right kidney corresponding to embedded part of space-taking lesion. Beak-shaped contour of kidney parenchyma.' Reprinted with permission from *Angiography* by H.L. Abrams (1961)'. Published by Little, Brown and Co., Boston

Figure 2. Penguin with prominent beak

BEATEN SILVER (BEATEN BRASS) PATTERN

Leo Davidoff[1], in 1936, studied the skull roentgenograms of nearly 2500 normal individuals in an attempt to understand the significance of the appearance of the convolutional markings upon the inner table of the skull. This work was done at the Neurological Institute in New York. The patients had an age range from 3 months to 18 years. The 'appearance of patchy areas of diminished density in the roentgenograms of the skull in certain cases is a matter of frequent experience. These areas are assumed to be the result of impressions of the cerebral convolutions upon the inner table of the skull, and when accompanied by pressure atrophy of the sella turcica or separation of the cranial sutures, or both, are indications of increased intracranial pressure. When the intracranial pressure is great, these markings may resemble beaten silver.'[1] (Figure 1). He emphasized that this appearance could be normal in growing children who did not have any other evidence of increased intracranial pressure. The presence of other signs of increased intracranial pressure was most important.

The beaten silver (beaten brass) pattern should be distinguished from lückenschädel[2] (lacunar skull) described by Gottfried Engstler (Pädiatrischen Klinik-Graz). Lacunar skull is seen in young infants (< 6 months) who have meningomyelocele, meningocele or encephalocele. It is a manifestation of the defective development of membranous bone and, therefore, is not related to the degree of increased intracranial pressure. The changes of lückenschädel are usually most pronounced in the parietal bones.

Silver is a precious metal, especially to the radiologist and to his film-making process. 'Silver ornaments and decorations have been found in royal tombs dating back as far as 4000 BC.'[3]

Brass is an 'alloy of copper and zinc, of historical and enduring importance because of its hardness and workability. The earliest brass, called calamine brass, dates to Neolithic times'[4] (Figure 2).

References

1. Davidoff, L.M. (1936). Convolutional digitations seen in the roentgenograms of immature human skulls. *Bull. Neurol. Inst. NY*, 5, 61–71

2. Engstler, G. (1905). Ueber den 'Lückenschädel' Neugeborener und seine Beziehung zur Spina Bifida. *Arch. Kinderheilkd.*, 40, 322–9

3. Silver. In *The New Encyclopaedia Britannica*, 1990, 15th edn., Vol. 10, p. 815. (Chicago: Encyclopaedia Britannica Inc.)

4. Brass. In *The New Encyclopedia Britannica*, 1990, 15th edn, Vol. 2, p. 480. (Chicago: Encyclopedia Britannica Inc.)

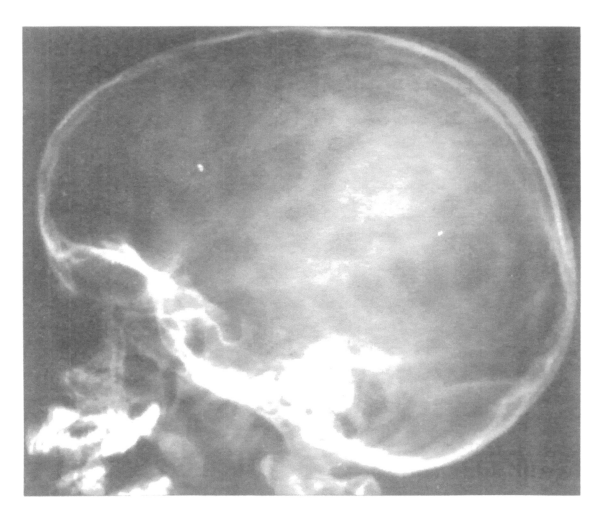

Figure 1. 'Skull X-ray of 7-year-old child'[1] showing beaten silver or brass pattern. Reprinted from Davidoff[1]. Convolutional digitations seen in the roentgenograms of immature human skulls. *Bull. Neurol. Inst. NY*, **5**, 61–71

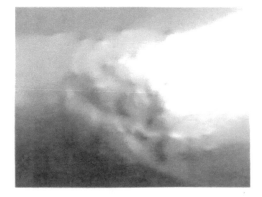

Figure 2. Hammer-beaten brass

BLADE OF GRASS (FLAME OR 'V') SIGN

The lytic phase of Paget's disease has characteristic appearances in the skull (osteoporosis circumscripta) and in the long bones (blade of grass, flame or V shape). Sir James Brailsford[1] (The Queen's Hospital, London), in the second edition of his textbook and in various papers, described the lytic process extending up or down the shaft of a long bone, with its sharply defined border, as V-shaped (Figure 1). 'When the disease affects the long bones and this is particularly noticeable in the tibia, the affected segment is sharply cut off from the normal ... The line of demarcation between the normal and the abnormal is usually V-shaped and sharply defined.'[2] Thomas Fairbank[3] said in 1950, 'The diagnostic value of the pointed extremity of the changes in the shaft of a long bone has been appreciated for many years, attention being called to it, we believe, by the late Professor S.G. Shattock [London].' Other terms including 'flame shaped' and 'blade of grass' have also been used to describe this appearance. The blade of grass terminology seems to be preferred today. This is a very reliable sign of Paget's disease (Figure 2). For acute, rapidly progressive forms, the term halisteresis was also used in Brailsford's day.

Grass is any of the many low, green, non-woody plants belonging to the grass family (Poaceae) (Figure 3). There are approximately 6000 to 10,000 species in the family[4].

References
1. Brailsford, J.F. (1935). *The Radiology of Bones and Joints*, 2nd edn. (London: J & A Churchill)

2. Brailsford, J.F. (1938). Paget's disease of bone, its frequency, diagnosis, and complications. *Br. J. Radiol.*, 2, 507–32

3. Fairbank, H.A.T. (1950). Paget's disease. *J. Bone Joint Surg.*, 32B, 253–65

4. Bews, J.W. (1929). *The World's Grasses*, pp. 1–34. (London: Longmans, Green & Co.)

Figure 1. 'Paget's disease of shaft of long bone.' Reprinted from Brailsford[2]. Paget's disease of bone. *Br. J. Radiol.*, 1938, **2**, 507–32, with permission of the British Institute of Radiology

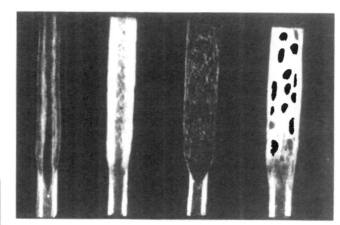

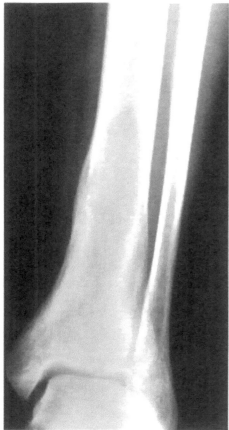

Figure 2. Radiograph showing blade of grass appearance in the tibia (author's case)

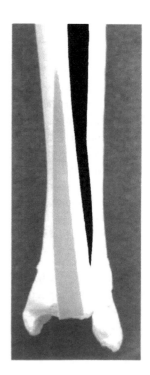

Figure 3. Tibia with super-imposed blade of grass

BOOT-SHAPED HEART (COEUR EN SABOT)

Sir William Osler[1] (1849–1919) attributed the term 'coeur en sabot,' used to describe the shape of the heart in cases of tetralogy of Fallot, to Henri Vaquez and E. Bordet. 'The most characteristic roentgen-ray features are the relatively small size of the left ventricle and the great hypertrophy of the right ventricle, which frequently curves around the smaller left chamber from below, rising upward like the tip of a sabot (Vaquez and Bordet), and giving rise to the descriptive term 'coeur en sabot', which is characteristic of the more pronounced cases associated with ventricular septal defect and dextroposition of the aorta.'[1] Vaquez (1860–1936) was a professor of the Faculty of Medicine in Paris and Bordet (1888–1925) was the chief of the laboratory. In Vaquez and Bordet's 1920 book[2], *The Heart and the Aorta,* the term is actually used in the discussion of 'Simple Stenosis of the Pulmonary Artery; The orthodiagraphic tracing ... presents the characteristic form known as 'en sabot': the heart apex is pushed outward and elevated'[2] (Figure 1). The term is not used in cases of pulmonary stenosis with interventricular communication, although these are two of the features of Fallot's tetralogy. Indeed, the authors did not mention their countryman, Etienne Fallot (1850–1911), even though his description of the four cardinal features of the cyanotic congenital heart disorder that now bears his name appeared in 1888[3]. Despite the apparent misappropriation by Osler, the term is now firmly associated with the shape of the cardiac silhouette seen in patients with the tetralogy of Fallot (Figure 2).

'From the earliest Oriental civilizations of Egypt and Mesopotamia come our sandal, shoe and boot. It is to the Theban frescoes painted on the walls of tombs in the fifteenth and nineteenth centuries before Christ that we go for the oldest pictures of the craft of shoemaking.'[4] The sabot was a heavy wooden work shoe or boot worn by European peasants, especially in France and the Low Countries (Figure 3). Wooden shoes were first mentioned in the Netherlands in the 1420s[5].

References

1. Osler, W. (1925). *Modern Medicine*, Vol. 4, p. 739. (Philadelphia: Lea & Febiger)

2. Vaquez, H. and Bordet, E. (1920). *The Heart and the Aorta*, translated from the 2nd French edn. Translated by Honeij, J.A. and Macy, J., p. 123. (New Haven: Yale University Press)

3. Fallot, E.(1888). Contribution à l'anatomie pathologique de la maladie bleue (cyanose cardiaque). *Marseille Médical*, 25, 418–20

4. Wilcox, R.T. (1948). *The Mode in Footwear*, pp. 2–3. (New York: Charles Scribner's Sons)

5. Noorlander, H. (1978). *Wooden Shoes, their Makers and their Wearers*, pp. 6–7. (Zutphen: Netherlands Open-Air Museum)

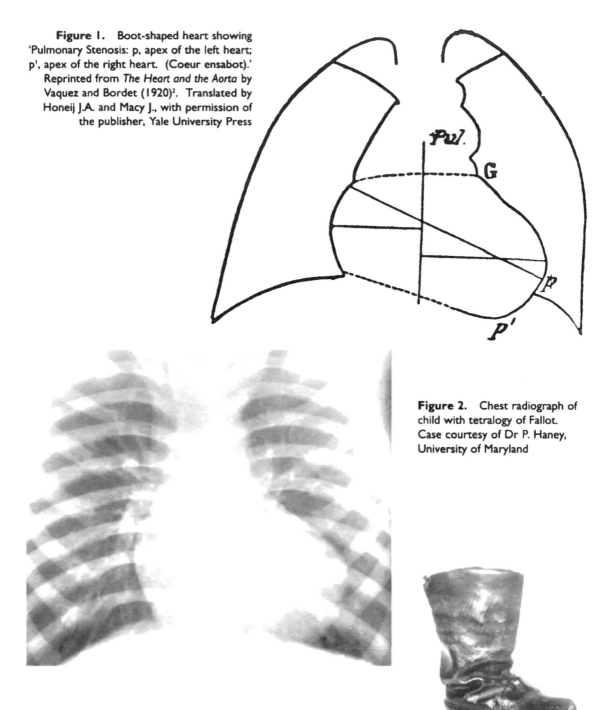

Figure 1. Boot-shaped heart showing 'Pulmonary Stenosis: p, apex of the left heart; p', apex of the right heart. (Coeur ensabot).' Reprinted from *The Heart and the Aorta* by Vaquez and Bordet (1920)[2]. Translated by Honeij J.A. and Macy J., with permission of the publisher, Yale University Press

Figure 2. Chest radiograph of child with tetralogy of Fallot. Case courtesy of Dr P. Haney, University of Maryland

Figure 3. Wooden shoe (sabot) with high leather boot leg. Photograph courtesy of Nederlands Openluchtmuseum, Arnhem, Netherlands

BOWLER HAT SIGN

Visualization and recognition of small polyps in the gastrointestinal tract, especially in the colon, have always been a challenge for radiologists. James Youker (University of California, San Francisco) and Sölve Welin[1] (University of Lund, Sweden) reported a new sign, that would help to do just that, at the fiftieth annual meeting of the Radiological Society of North America in 1964. Many articles were written in the 1950s and early 1960s discussing the relationship between polyps and colon cancer. Differentiating polyps from other filling defects on an air-contrast barium enema became very important and remains so today. Youker and Welin[1] analyzed more than 21 000 air-contrast examinations and emphasized two signs, the bowler hat and the target, in their report. For sessile polyps, 'An analogy can be made to a bowler hat in which the coated body of the polyp represents the crown and the barium around the base the brim.'[1] (Figure 1). Visualization of a target sign identified a stalked polyp, 'When the roentgen beam passes parallel to the long axis of the barium-coated pedicle, it appears as a small circle within the larger barium circle, surrounding the main body of the polyp.'[1]

The bowler hat, as a clothing item, originated in England in 1850. It was designed by the hatters James and George Lock at number 6 St James Street, London. William Coke II, later the Earl of Leicester, had commissioned a new hat for the protection of his gamekeepers' heads as they rode through his wooded estate. The Locks sent their design across the Thames to the hatmakers Thomas and William Bowler who were their chief suppliers and whose name became synonymous with the new hat[2]. The hat was quickly adopted by the middle class people of the time. It was made famous by many entertainers including Charlie Chaplin, Laurel and Hardy, and by the artist René Magritte. One of Magritte's paintings of a bowler hat is shown as Figure 2.

References

1. Youker, J.E. and Welin, S. (1965). Differentiation of true polypoid tumors of the colon from extraneous material: a new roentgen sign. *Radiology*, 84, 610–15

2. Robinson, F.M. (1993). *The Man in the Bowler Hat*, pp. 5–16. (Chapel Hill, NC: University of North Carolina Press)

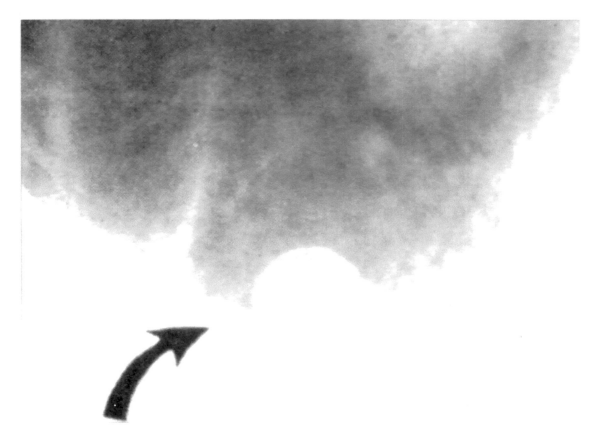

Figure 1. 'Intermediate type of polyp with 'hat sign'.' Reprinted from Youker and Welin[1]. Differentiation of true polypoid tumors of the colon from extraneous material. *Radiology*, 1965, **84**, 610–15, with permission of the RSNA

Figure 2. *The Fright Stopper* by René Magritte. Copyright 1995 C. Herscovici, Brussels/Artists Rights Society (ARS), New York

BULLET SHAPED (BULLET-NOSE) VERTEBRAE

One of the distinct, and sometimes distinguishing, features of the many forms of dwarfism is the appearance of the vertebral bodies. Vertebral body shapes can include flattened rectangles, round forms and those with pointed projections from one surface or another. In achondroplasia the lateral view of the lumbar vertebrae shows that they have a shape resembling a large- caliber blunt-nose bullet (Figure 1). John Caffey[1] (Babies Hospital, New York) used the term bullet-nose deformity to describe this appearance in his 1958 article on achondroplasia. This paper was an in depth review of the radiographic features of achondroplasia in the pelvis and lumbosacral spine. 'Regional under-growth of the ventral ends of some lumbar vertebral bodies appears to be responsible for their wedging ventrad and the pinching of their ventral ends into rounded bullet-nose deformities. In our achondroplastic patients, these deformities have been found only after the first year of life; similar deformities have been present in cretins and gargoyles during the first months of life.'[1]

Other characteristic spinal and vertebral abnormalities in achondroplasia include spinal stenosis (due to narrowing of the interpediculate distance and short pedicles) and scalloping of the posterior vertebral body.

The first projectiles fired from a weapon were probably stones shot from a mortar. These weapons probably originated about AD 1240, in north Africa. Cannons appeared around AD 1330 and hand-held firearms with bullets were developed 50–100 years later[2] Figure 2 shows three types of modern handgun ammunition.

References

1. Caffey, J. (1958). Achondroplasia of pelvis and lumbosacral spine. *Am J. Roentgenol.*, 80, 449–57

2. Held, R. (1957). *The Age of Firearms*, p. 18. (New York: Harper & Brothers Publishers)

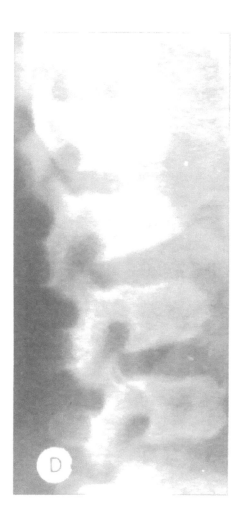

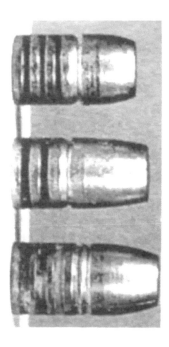

Figure 1. 'Smallness and pinching of the ventral ends of the first and second lumbar bodies into rounded bullet-nosed deformities.' Reprinted from Caffey[1]. Achondroplasia of pelvis and lumbosacral spine. *Am. J. Roentgenol.*, **80**, 449–57 with the permission of the ARRS

Figure 2. Hand gun ammunition

BUTTERFLY AND BAT'S WING SHADOW

Herrnheiser and Hinson[1] (London Chest Hospital) credit Curtis Nessa and Leo Rigler[2] with the term 'butterfly density' and Hodson[3] with the term 'bat's wing shadow' as descriptions of the chest radiographic appearance of pulmonary edema (Figures 1 and 2). These authors may have been the first to put these terms in the printed literature, however, they say in their articles that the 'classical roentgenologic appearance *has been* [my italics] described as a butterfly-shaped ... density'[2] and that a 'search in the literature for reference to the 'bat'swing' lesion gives disappointing results. It appears to have become accepted as an established abnormality without its natural history and significance being fully defined.'[3] The latter statement seems to refer to both the term and the disease process.

Nonetheless, Nessa and Rigler[2] (University of Minnesota), did study 110 patients who had died with moderate or severe pulmonary edema. All 110 patients had postmortem examinations. They emphasized the variety of patterns that could be seen in addition to the classical 'butterfly' with central air-space opacity and a more normal peripheral zone. Today we attribute this pattern to more efficient lymphatic clearance of fluid from the periphery of the lung.

Hodson[3] (University College Hospital, London) reported six cases of pulmonary edema to re-emphasize the radiographic bat's wing pattern and the associated condition since they were 'More widely recognized perhaps in America than in [his] country.'

Butterflies are in the class Insecta, order Lepidoptera (Figure 3). They have been found in fossils dated 100 to 130 million-years-old. Bats belong to the class Mammalia, order Chiroptera (Figure 4). The steps in the evolution of flight in bats and the development of their 'wings' are still debated[4].

References
1. Herrnheiser, G. and Hinson, K.F.W. (1954). An anatomical explanation of the formation of butterfly shadows. *Thorax*, 9, 198–210
2. Nessa, C.B. and Rigler, L.G. (1941). The roentgenological manifestations of pulmonary edema. *Radiology*, 37, 35–46
3. Hodson, C.J. (1950). Pulmonary œdema and the 'bat's wing' shadow. *J. Fac. Radiol. (London)*, 1, 176–86
4. Padian, K. (1987). A comparative phylogenetic and functional approach to the origin of vertebrate flight. In Fenton, M.B., Racey, P. and Rayner, J.M.V. (eds.) *Recent Advances in the Study of Bats*, pp. 3–22. (Cambridge: Cambridge University Press)

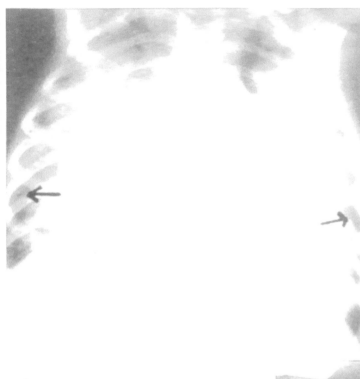

Figure 1. 'Typical pulmonary edema from cardiac failure. Note the bilateral, symmetrical, butterfly-shaped densities with the relatively clear periphery (arrows)' Reprinted from Nessa and Rigler[2]. The roentgenological manifestations of pulmonary edema. *Radiology*, 1941, **37**, 35–46, with permission of the RSNA

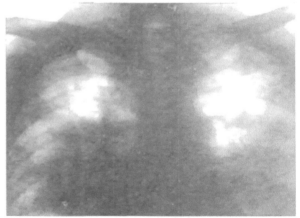

Figure 2. 'After probable attack of left heart failure. Widespread bilateral 'bat's wing' shadows with moderate congestion but no definite basal edema.' Reprinted from Hodson[3]. Pulmonary oedema and the 'bat's wing' shadow. *J. Fac. Radiol. (London)*, 1950, **1**, 176–86, with permission of the publisher

Figure 3. A butterfly

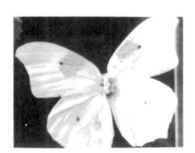

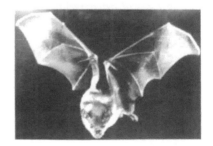

Figure 4. A bat on the wing

BUTTON SEQUESTRUM

United States Army Colonel Paul Wells[1] wrote about the button sequestrum in 1956. He described four patients with eosinophilic granulomas affecting their skulls who were seen at Letterman Army Hospital in San Francisco. In each case, a central sequestrum resembling a button was evident on the plain-film radiographs (Figure 1). 'Among the many articles which describe this lesion, however, only one has specifically called attention to the rather characteristic sequestrum produced in some of these cases. This sequestrum appears as a 'button' of intact bone in the center of a circular area of destruction.'[1] He referred to a 1946 paper by four other Army officers, also from Letterman Army Hospital, that discussed nine cases of eosinophilic granuloma[2]. One of the cases in the earlier article had sequestra found at operation but they could not be seen on the preoperative roentgenogram and there was no discussion of sequestra in that report.

Eosinophilic granuloma of bone was the term used to describe this disease entity, in 1940, by Louis Lichtenstein and Henry Jaffe[3] (Hospital for Joint Diseases, New York). Sadao Otani and Joseph Ehrlich[4] (Mount Sinai Hospital and Lebanon Hospital, New York), in the same year, used the term solitary granuloma of bone. The current term is Langerhans cell histiocytosis (LCH). Sequestra seen on radiologic imaging studies are not specific for LCH. They may also be seen in cases of osteomyelitis, primary lymphoma of bone, and in some fibrous tumors, classically fibrosarcoma[5].

Buttons date back to the ancient Greeks and Etruscans who fastened their tunics with them. Commonly used buttons then were made of bone

or wood[6]. Buttons made of bone were still common in the first half of this century and are occasionally found on shirts and suits manufactured today. The bone button shown in Figure 2 is from a 'union suit' set of long underwear *circa* 1920.

References
1. Wells, P.O. (1956). The button sequestrum of eosinophilic granuloma of the skull. *Radiology*, 67, 746–7

2. Hamilton, J.B., Barner, J.L., Kennedy, P.C. and McCort, J.J. (1946). The osseous manifestations of eosinophilic granuloma: report of nine cases. *Radiology*, 47, 445–56

3. Lichtenstein, L. and Jaffe, H.L. (1940). Eosinophilic granuloma of bone, with report of a case. *Am. J. Pathol.*, 16, 595–604

4. Otani, S. and Ehrlich, J.C. (1940). Solitary granuloma of bone simulating primary neoplasm. *Am. J. Pathol.*, 16, 479–90

5. Mulligan, M.E. and Kransdorf, M.J. (1993). Sequestra in primary lymphoma of bone: prevalence and radiologic features. *Am. J. Roentgenol.*, 160, 1245–8

6. Button. In *The New Encyclopaedia Britannica*, 1990, 15th edn., Vol. 2, p. 688. (Chicago: Encyclopaedia Britannica Inc.)

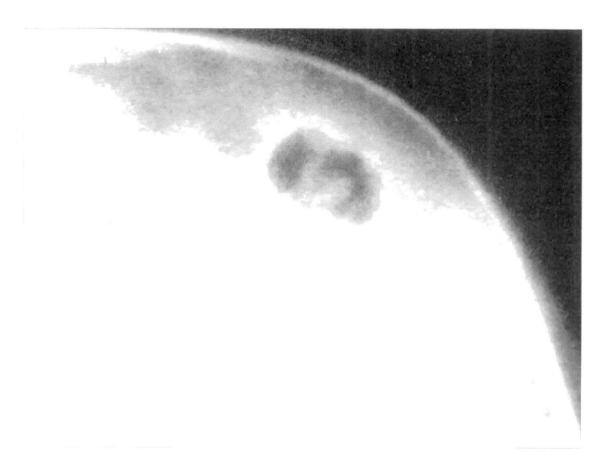

Figure 1. 'The osteolytic lesion in the right parietal bone involves both tables of the calvarium and contains a 'button' of bone.' Reprinted from Wells[1]. The button sequestrum of eosinophilic granuloma of the skull. *Radiology*, 1956, **67**, 746–7, with the permission of the RSNA

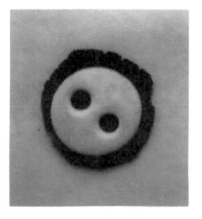

Figure 2. A button made of bone

CAMALOTE (WATERLILY) SIGN

The sign of the camalote was firmly established, in the English literature, in 1949 by Fainsinger's report[1] from Johannesburg. He described the typical findings in a 54-year-old man. Camalotes are waterlilies whose floating fronds are brought to mind by the floating membranes of a collapsed hydatid endocyst as seen on a chest radiograph (Figure 1).

Parasitic hydatid disease was common in South Africa at the time of Fainsinger's report because of the large sheep-raising industry. Before the lung cysts, caused by this disease, collapsed by communicating with a bronchus, there was nothing unique about their X-ray appearance that allowed a specific diagnosis to be made. Recognition of the sign of the camalote was pathognomonic for hydatid disease. Fainsinger[1] said that South American writers had likened the X-ray appearance to that of the camalote, although he cites no one specifically. According to Víctor Armand Ugón in his book, *El Torax Quirurgico* (The Surgical Thorax), the South American who first described the sign of the camalote was Lagos García of Uruguay[2]. 'What is truly pathognomonic is the sign of the camalote of Lagos García that appears in the image as an air–fluid level in the cyst. It consists of a crumpled line that is seen swimming over the liquid; other times it manifests itself like a bubble or an arcing line that emerges from the liquid portion, or like an irregularity from the fluid. The sign of the camalote when found carefully has diagnostic value in considering the hydatid pyopneumocyst. The sign described by Lagos García is determined by the withdrawn germinative layer, floating on the liquid contained in the cyst cavity.'[2]

Waterlilies are any of the freshwater plants of the family Nymphaeaceae. They have rounded floating waxy-coated leaves on long stalks[3] (Figure 2).

References

1. Fainsinger, M.H. (1949). Pulmonary hydatid disease: the sign of the camalote. *S. Afr. Med. J.*, 23, 723

2. Armand Ugón, V. (1938). *El Torax Quirurgico*, p. 310. (Montevideo: Editorial Libertad)

3. Waterlily. In *The New Encyclopaedia Britannica*, 1990, 15th edn., Vol. 12, p. 516. (Chicago: Encyclopaedia Britannica Inc.)

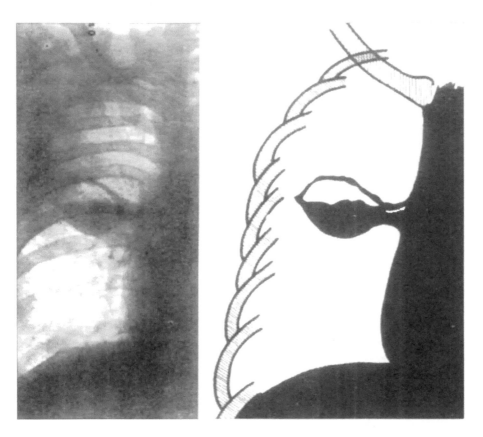

Figure 1. Chest X-ray with clarifying diagram showing a hydatid cyst with the sign of the camalote. Modified from *El Torax Quirurgico* by Armand Ugón[2] (1938)

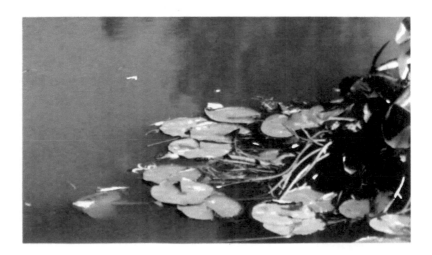

Figure 2. Waterlily pond, Monet's home, Giverny, France

CARPENTER'S LEVEL SIGN

One of the most important things a radiologist must do when interpreting a barium enema is to distinguish polyps from air bubbles and other filling defects. This applies to both solid-column and double-column barium enemas. John Mulloy and Randall Scott[1] (University of Tennessee, Memphis) have aided us in this task with regard to the solid-column barium enema, by their recent description of the 'carpenter's level sign'[1]. When a filling defect maintains a central position on a solid-column barium enema, with views at 90° (e.g. supine and lateral), a carpenter's level air bubble sign is present (Figure 1). As in a carpenter's level (Figure 2), the filling defect in the column is an air bubble seeking the highest point in the column. After discussing the movement of an air bubble verses a polyp, during a film interpreting session, the authors devised a model that would simulate the *in vivo* findings (Mulloy, personal communication). 'An air bubble and a sessile polyp can occupy similar positions within the image of the colon [on supine or prone films] if the polyp is located centrally on the anterior or posterior wall. When the model was turned 90°, the air bubble was seen to hold its central position in the highest point of the column, whereas the polyp moved with the direction of rotation to display a profile view from what was then the lateral wall.'[1] The authors then confirmed their experimental results during barium enema examination of patients.

This sign is especially useful in elderly debilitated patients undergoing a single-contrast barium enema when a double-contrast barium enema with its requisite upright views is not possible.

The simple carpenter's level with a string plumb bob, the Roman libella, has existed since the times of Lucretius, Pliny and Varro (AD first century). The 'spirit level' (filled with alcohol) was invented by Thevenot in 1666. It did not become popular until the Industrial Revolution (1760–1850 in Britain) when it could be mass produced[2].

References
1. Mulloy, J.P. and Scott, R.L. (1994). Differentiating colonic polyps from air bubbles on barium enema: the 'carpenter's level sign'. *Am. J. Roentgenol.*, 163, 84–6
2. Mercer, H.C. (1960). *Ancient Carpenters' Tools*, pp. 65–6. (Doylestown, PA: Bucks County Historical Society)

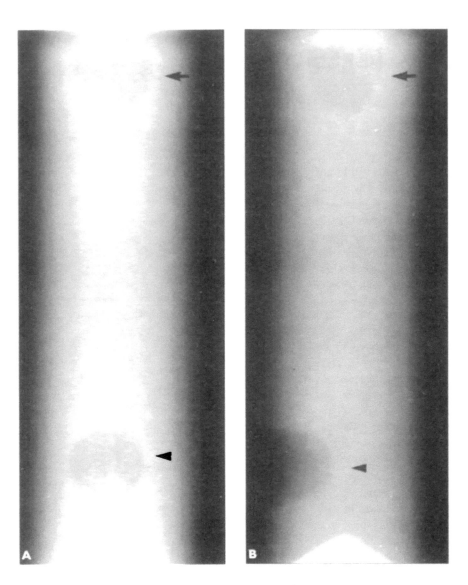

Figure 1. 'Comparison of radiographic appearance of an air bubble and a sessile polyp in perpendicular views. A, an air bubble (arrow) and a sessile polyp (a gumdrop in this model; arrowhead) can produce a nearly identical appearance on radiographs. B, after model is rotated 90 degrees, simulated polyp (arrowhead) is seen in profile projecting from lateral wall. Air bubble (arrow) has maintained central highest point – a positive 'carpenter's level sign'.' Reprinted from Mulloy and Scott[1]. Differentiating colonic polyps from air bubbles on barium enema: the 'carpenter's level sign'. *Am. J. Roentgenol.*, 1994, **163**, 84–6, with the permission of the ARRS

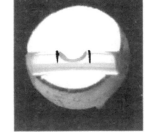

Figure 2. A carpenter's level

CELERY-STICK (CELERY STALK) METAPHYSIS

This term likens the long bone radiographic appearance of alternating vertical dense and lucent metaphyseal striations (Figure 1), caused by rubella infection, to the 'ridges' (actually phloem and xylem channels) in a celery stalk (Figure 2). A rubella epidemic in the United States, in the spring and summer of 1964, generated many scientific papers on the clinical and roentgenologic manifestations of rubella embryopathy which were foremost in the minds and practices of many physicians at that time.

The term, celery stick, first appeared in an article by Hugh Williams and Lewis Carey[1] (St Joseph's Hospital and Children's Hospital, St Paul, Minnesota) published in the *American Journal of Roentgenology* in May 1966[1]. They discussed seven cases in the paper stating 'Because of the current widespread epidemic of rubella in this country and the frequency of associated roentgenologic findings, it is imperative that every radiologist be familiar with the roentgenologic features of rubella embryopathy.'[1] The celery-stick metaphyseal striations were just one of the several skeletal findings they discussed in addition to the various cardiovascular and pulmonary findings reported. 'The principal changes occurred in the metaphyses of the long bones, particularly the distal femurs, and consisted of alternating dense and radiolucent longitudinal striations. These produce a celery-stick appearance in the affected metaphyses.'[1]

Celery *(Apium graveolens)* is a herb of the family Apiaceae. It is native to the Mediterranean area and the middle East. Celery was used as a flavoring by the Greeks and Romans and as a medicine by the ancient Chinese[2].

References

1. Williams, H.J. and Carey, L.S. (1966). Rubella embryopathy: roentgenologic features. *Am. J. Roentgenol.*, 97, 92–9

2. Celery. In *The New Encyclopaedia Britannica*, 1990, 15th edn., Vol. 3, p.9. (Chicago: Encyclopaedia Britannica Inc.)

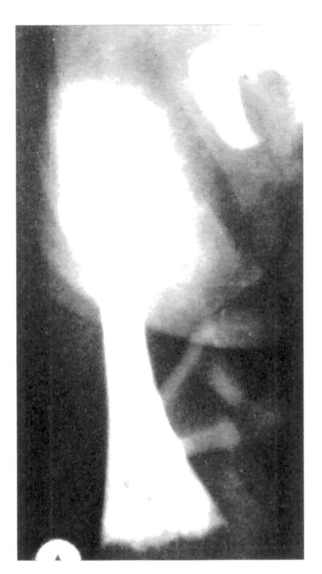

Figure 1. 'Alternating radiolucent and dense longitudinal metaphyseal striations produce a 'celery stick' appearance.' Reprinted from Williams and Carey[1]. Rubella embryopathy: roentgenologic features. *Am. J. Roentgenol.*, 1966, **97**, 92–9, with the permission of the ARRS

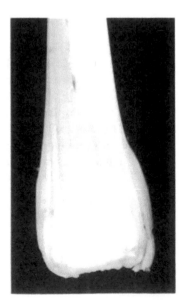

Figure 2. A stick of celery

CLOVERLEAF SKULL

Kleeblattschädel is the German term used, by Karl Holtermüller and Hans Wiedemann[1] in 1960, to describe a cloverleaf-shaped deformity of the skull. They described one case of their own and reviewed the findings in 12 other cases. These authors used the term kleeblattschädel (cloverleaf skull) to describe a well-defined syndrome. The main features were: '(1) cloverleaf deformity, the cardinal symptom; (2) facial malformations involving the orbits, nose and upper maxilla; (3) occasionally, chondrodysplastic changes affecting the limbs and the spine; (4) severe hydrocephalus; and (5) poor prognosis due to progressive intracranial hypertension.'[2] A cloverleaf-shape of the skull (Figure 1) can be seen in several other conditions, especially thanatophoric dysplasia and the craniostenoses[2]. 'The deformity is due to severe alterations in skull development with premature synostosis of some cranial sutures associated with marked hydrocephalus, resulting in a striking bulging of the head upward in the region of the anterior fontanel and laterally in the temporal regions, the latter forming the lateral lobes of the cloverleaf.'[2]

Clover or trefoil is the common name for plants in the genus *Trifolium* (family Leguminosae). There are about 250 species of clover. Clover leaves usually come in threes (Figure 2), but occasional four-lobed leaves are found. Four-leaved clovers are thought to be good-luck charms. Clover is 'unexcelled in furnishing forage and fodder to domestic animals, and unequalled in the renovating influences which they exert upon land.'[3]

References
1. Holtermüller, K. and Wiedemann, H.R. (1960). Kleeblattschädel. *Med. Maschr.*, 14, 439

2. Iannaccone, G. and Gerlini, G. (1974). The so-called 'cloverleaf skull syndrome'. *Pediatr. Radiol.*, 2, 175–84

3. Shaw, T. (1906). *Clovers and How to Grow Them*, p. 1. (New York: Orange Judd Co.)

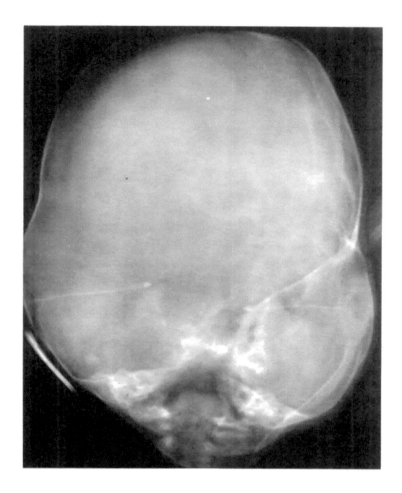

Figure 1. Skull radiograph showing cloverleaf deformity. Case courtesy of Dr A. Campbell, University of Maryland

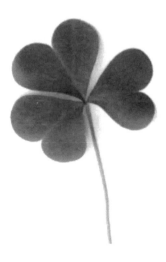

Figure 2. A cloverleaf

COBBLESTONE PATTERN

Regional ileitis was the name given by Burrill Crohn, Leon Ginzburg and Gordon Oppenheimer[1] (Mount Sinai Hospital, New York) in 1932 to the pathologic and clinical entity they described that has become known as Crohn's disease. Their report of 14 cases included a detailed pathologic study of resected specimens from 13 of the patients. Regarding the pathologic changes in this inflammatory disease of the terminal ileum, they said, 'The characteristic, fully developed hypertrophic process is, as a rule, limited to the distal 25 to 35 cm of the terminal ileum ... the normal intestinal folds are distorted and broken up by the destructive ulcerative process and rounded and blunted by edema, giving a bullous structure to the mucosal aspect of the intestine, or frequently a cobblestone appearance of the surface of the mucosa may result.'[1] They did not make use of the cobblestone term in the short discussion of their roentgenographic observations. Only one radiograph was reproduced in the article, it does not show a cobblestone pattern. This gross pathologic appearance was subsequently transferred into the language of radiologists who recognized the same pattern on barium studies done on subsequent patients (Figure 1). There are very few other conditions which cause a similar cobblestone pattern in the terminal ileum thus making it a useful sign.

A cobblestone is 'a water-worn rounded stone, such as is used for paving.'[2] Cobblestone streets can still be found in most European cities and in some of the older cities in the United States (Figure 2).

References

1. Crohn, B.B, Ginzburg, L. and Oppenheimer, G.D. (1932). Regional ileitis – a pathologic and clinical entity. *J. Am. Med. Assoc.*, 99, 1323–9

2. Simpson, J. and Weiner, E. (eds.) *Oxford English Dictionary*, 1989, 2nd edn, Vol. 3, p. 402. (Oxford: Clarendon Press)

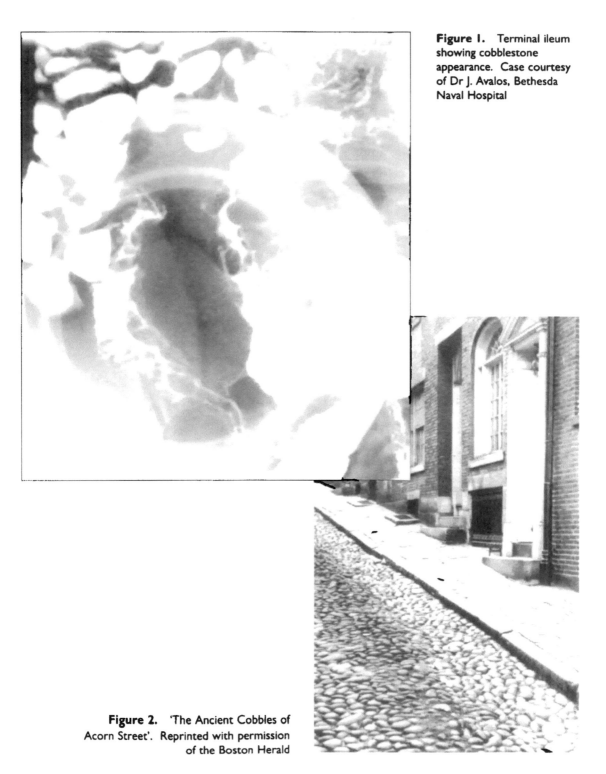

Figure 1. Terminal ileum showing cobblestone appearance. Case courtesy of Dr J. Avalos, Bethesda Naval Hospital

Figure 2. 'The Ancient Cobbles of Acorn Street'. Reprinted with permission of the Boston Herald

COBRA HEAD (SNAKE HEAD) URETER

Thomas Canigiani[1] (Röntgeninstitutes des Kaiser Fronz-Josef-Spitales in Wein) is said by some to have made the first roentgenographic diagnosis of a ureterocele[2]. However, it was John Hellström, who reported 15 cases in the 1937 *Acta Radiologica*, who described the schlangenkopf (snake head or cobra head) picture seen by urography as pathognomonic for the presence of a ureterocele[3] (Figure 1). He emphasized that failure to see the snake head did not exclude the possibility of a ureterocele. The 'cobra head' represents the dilated terminal portion of the ureter as seen by excretory urography or by cystoscopy. The dilatation may be caused by an abnormally small ureteral orifice or abnormal emptying due to an ectopic position.

Ureteroceles may generally be divided into two types, simple and ectopic. A stenotic or abnormally small orifice is the usual explanation for the formation of a simple ureterocele. The abnormal insertion of the ectopic ureter into the bladder wall is said to account for the ureterocele in this type. True ureteroceles must be distinguished from pseudoureteroceles. Pseudoureteroceles may be caused by inflammatory or neoplastic processes that cause obstruction of the ureteral orifice.

The Indian cobra *(Naja naja)* averages 4–5 feet in length and is found on most of the Indian subcontinent and in Sri Lanka. When the cobra's hood is spread, a distinct marking is evident that is usually described by herpetologists as a pair of spectacles[4]. To the genitourinary tract specialist, this hood marking might more closely resemble the two kidneys with their draining ureters rather than a pair of spectacles (Figure 2). This certainly makes the cobra head or cobra hood terminology even more appropriate for the radiographic appearance of a ureterocele.

References

1. Canigiani, T. (1932–3). Ein Fall von cystischer Dilatation des vesicalen Ureterendes *Z. Urol. Chir.*, 36, 172

2. Williams, E.R. (1936). Ureterocele. *Br. J. Radiol.*, 9, 59–66

3. Hellström, J. (1937). Zur Kenntnis der isolierten Dilatation des Pelvinen oder juxtavesikalen Harnleiterabschnittes. *Acta Radiol.*, 18, 141–56

4. Ditmars, R.L. (1931). *Snakes of the World*, pp. 155–6. (New York: Macmillan Publishing Co. Inc.)

5. Thompson, G.J. and Kelalis, P.P. (1964). Ureterocele. *J. Urol.*, 91, 488–92

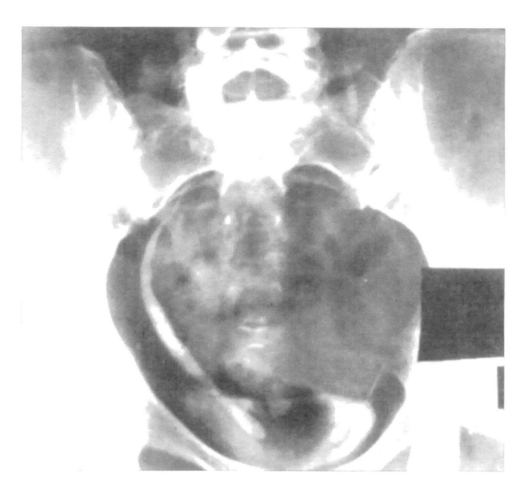

Figure 1. 'Bilateral ureteroceles
show typical cobra-head deformity.'
Reprinted from Thompson and Kelalis[5].
Ureterocele. *J. Urol.*, 1964, **91**, 488–92,
with permission of Williams & Wilkins

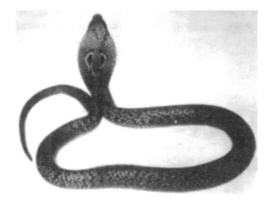

Figure 2. Indian cobra *(Naja naja).*
Reprinted from *Snakes of the World* by
Ditmars (1931)[4], with permission of The
New York Zoological Society.© NYZS/The
Wildlife Conservation Society

CODFISH (FISH) VERTEBRA

This biconcave deformity of the vertebral endplates is seen in many disorders (Figure 1). Donald Resnick[1] (University of California and VA Medical Center, San Diego) lists osteoporosis, osteomalacia, hyperparathyroidism and Paget's disease among them.

The origin of this term 'is obscure, but it was probably introduced by a Boston radiologist who, influenced by provincial pisciculture and local dietary customs, used the species-specific phrase 'codfish vertebra'.'[2] Jack Reynolds[2] (University of Texas Southwestern), in his 1965 review article, stated that it 'was originally coined to describe the spinal changes which are most frequently observed in patients with senile osteoporosis.' He discussed its use in reference to the spinal changes in sickle-cell disease, although he considered this usage unfortunate. He lamented that 'while the two types of deformities differ, the shape of each bears some resemblance to the vertebra of a fish, and, as yet, no substitute form of descriptive imagery has been fashioned to succinctly indicate the unique qualities of this stigma of the hemoglobinopathy.'[2] (See 'Lincoln Log' sign).

The Atlantic cod *(Gadus morhua)* is one of about 60 species in the family Gadidae. This important source of food and liver oil is usually found in cold northern seas. These fish can be up to 6 feet in length and may weigh up to 200 pounds[3]. Vertebrae of codfish are indeed biconcave as is shown in the specimen radiograph (Figure 2).

References
1. Resnick, D.L. (1982). Fish vertebrae. *Arthritis Rheum.*, 25, 1073–7

2. Reynolds, J. (1965). A re-evaluation of the 'fish vertebra' sign in sickle cell hemoglobinopathy. *Am. J. Roentgenol.*, 97, 693–707

3. Jensen, A.C. (1972). *The Cod*, pp. 4–37. (New York: Thomas Y. Crowell Co.)

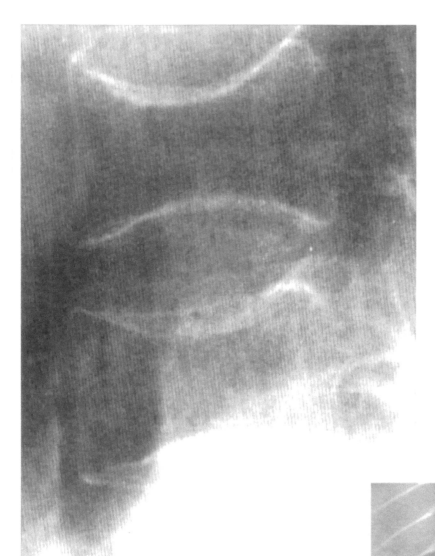

Figure 1. 'The centra of an elderly subject showing the classic biconcave contour of the sort commonly caused by osteoporosis for which the term 'fish vertebra deformity' was originally coined.' Reprinted from Reynolds[2] a re-evaluation of the 'fish verteba' sign in sickle cell hemoglobinopathy. *Am. J. Roentgenol.,* **97,** 693–707, with permission of the ARRS

Figure 2. Lateral radiograph of codfish's spine. Specimen radiograph by John Bode, Registered Radiologic Technologist (RRT)

CODMAN TRIANGLE (CODMAN ANGLE)

Reactive triangles of periosteal new bone formation (Figure 1) were pointed out by Hugo Ribbert[1] (Bonn University) in 1914. In bone tumors of central origin, he said that the elevation of the periosteum represented 'an area of newly formed non-tumor bone ... due to ... the adjacent expanding tumor mass.'[2]

Ernest Amory Codman[3] (1869–1940) was the principal driving force behind the organization of the Registry of Bone Sarcoma in the US (with help from James Ewing and Joseph Bloodgood). In 1920, at the request of the family of one of his bone tumor patients, he began the process of detailed data collection that led to the formation of the Registry. In his 1926 report on osteosarcoma he discussed the origin of the Registry and enumerated the 25 criteria used to establish a diagnosis of osteogenic sarcoma[3]. The first of the five X-ray criteria discussed concerned 'Combined central and subperiosteal involvement.' Regarding bone outside the cortex, he said, 'The little cuff of reactive bone of trumpet shape which surrounds the upper limit of the tumor appears in the X-ray as a triangular space on each side of the shaft under the uplifted periosteal edge. The presence of this is a sure indication of subperiosteal extracortical involvement. It represents the last line of defense of normal osteoblasts retreating in circular formation as the tumor advances under the periosteum' (Figure 2). For all he did to advance our knowledge of bone sarcomas, it is fitting that the periosteal triangle sign has come to bear his name. This sign is not specific for bone tumors since any process that causes periosteal elevation (e.g. infection, hemorrhage) may lead to the formation of a Codman triangle. Some prefer the term Codman angle when the short side along the edge of the extra osseous process is lucent.

Although the Egyptians and Babylonians are known to have had a working knowledge of geometry and triangles as early as 2000–3000 BC, they gave us 'no theoretical results, nor are any general rules of procedure given ...

It is to the Greeks that we turn in order to find the notion of a rigorous deductive proof, the method of developing the subject by an orderly sequence of theorems based upon definitions, axioms and postulates.'[4] The Greek Thales of Miletus (624–546 BC) is said to have 'established geometry as a deductive science.'[4] (Figure 3) Pythagoras (569–500 BC) and Euclid (fourth century BC) were two later Greek mathematicians who are perhaps more well known to geometry students.

References

1. Ribbert, H. (1914). *Geschwulstlehre für Aertze und Studierende.* (Bonn: Cohen)

2. Brunschwig, A. and Harmon, P.H. (1935). Studies in bone sarcoma. *Surg. Gynecol. Obstet.*, 60, 30–40

3. Codman, E.A. (1926). Registry of Bone Sarcoma. *Surg. Gynecol. Obstet.*, 42, 381–93

4. Scott, J.F (1958). *A History of Mathematics – From Antiquity to the Beginning of the Nineteenth Century,* pp. 1–33. (London: Taylor and Francis Ltd)

5. Codman, E.A. (1925). The nomenclature used by the Registry of Bone Sarcoma. *Am. J. Roentgenol.*, 13, 105–26

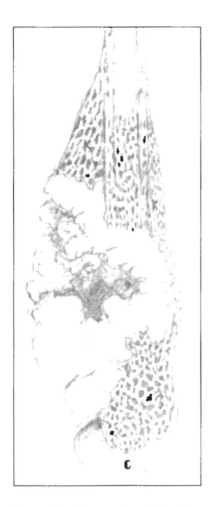

Figure 2. 'Registry #513. One sees not only the tumor developing radiating spicules outside of the cortex but an area of loss of density within the bone itself.'[3] A Codman triangle is evident at the proximal margin of the tumor along the anterior surface of the femur. Reprinted from Codman[5] The nomenclature used by the Registry of Bone Sarcoma. *Am. J. Roentgenol.*, **13**, 105–126, with permission of the ARRS

Figure 1. Diagram from Ribbert's work showing triangle of periosteal bone. Reprinted from *Geschwulstlehre für Aertze und Studierende* by Ribbert (1914)[1], published by Cohen

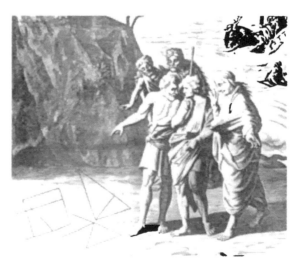

Figure 3. Aristippus shipwrecked on the shore at Rhodes observes geometric figures. Frontispiece to *Euclidis*. Oxford, 1703

COFFEE BEAN SIGN

Leo Rigler[1] (University of Minnesota) was one of the giants of gastrointestinal radiology. In a 1944 review of roentgen diagnosis of acute abdominal conditions, he mentions the 'coffee bean' as a useful sign of strangulating bowel obstruction saying, 'In many cases, the gas-filled bowel has taken on a characteristic 'coffee bean' appearance, the two loops being separated by a wide band of increased density, probably representing the edematous walls of the bowel with a small amount of fluid between them [Figure 1]. There is an unusually large accumulation of fluid within these isolated loops, and they remain relatively fixed, so that in the upright or lateral decubitus position the distended loops of bowel do not shift.'

The use of this sign and other signs was important since '[d]ifferentiation of simpel [simple] mechanical obstruction from a strangulation is of extreme importance, particularly with relationship to the application of therapy. While in simple mechanical obstruction, the application of conservative suction therapy may be the method of choice, such a procedure in the presence of a strangulation ... may result in a fatality directly attributable to the neglect of proper procedures.'[1] He originally used the term when describing cases of small bowel obstruction[2]. The term has also been applied to cases of large bowel obstruction, especially volvulus of the sigmoid colon.

'Nobody, today, would dispute that coffee [or bowel obstruction] is big [or important] business; in fact, after oil it is reckoned to be the most widely traded commodity in the world ... The coffee tree is indigenous to Ethiopia but the early history of its cultivation and the use of coffee as a beverage ... is centered on Arabia ... in the fifteenth century ...

[C]offee beans are the seeds of an evergreen shrub belonging to the family Rubiaceae and the genus *Coffea*.'[3] (Figure 2).

References

1. Rigler, L.G. (1944). Roentgen diagnosis of acute abdominal conditions: a review. *Bull. Univ. Minn. Hosp.*, 16, 120–37

2. Mellins, H.Z. and Rigler, L.G. (1954). The roentgen findings in strangulating obstructions of the small bowel. *Am. J. Roentgenol.*, 71, 404–15

3. Smith, A.W. (1985). In Clarke, R.J. and Macrae, R. (eds.) *Coffee*, Vol. 1, pp. 1–3. (London: Elsevier Applied Science Publishers)

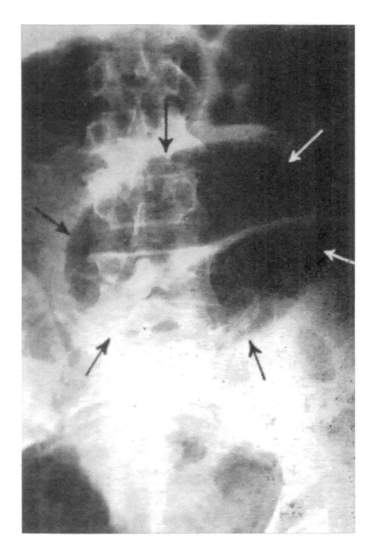

Figure 1. "Coffee bean' sign. Operation revealed a gas-distended, incarcerated loop, obstructed at two points by postoperative adhesions.' Reprinted from Mellins and Rigler[2] The roentgen findings in strangulating obstructions of the small bowel. *Am. J. Roentgenol.*, **71**, 404–15, with permission from the ARRS

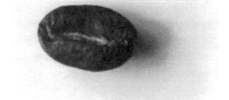

Figure 2. A coffee bean

COIN LESION

'Community and general hospital chest roentgeno-graphic surveys have resulted in the 'coin' lesions becoming a common and important problem,' so said William Ford and his surgical colleagues[1] from the University of Pittsburgh in 1956. They attributed the first report of a coin lesion of the lung (Figure 1) to Hans Chiari[2] in 1883. Their four criteria, for describing a pulmonary nodule as a coin lesion, are still largely valid today and are: '(1) a diameter between 1 and 4 cm [3 cm is the usual upper limit today], (2) a well-circumscribed tumor, (3) a lesion surrounded by lung, and (4) no evidence of major bronchial obstruction.' They chose a maximum diameter of 4 cm since that was the size of the largest United States coin, the silver dollar, at that time (Figure 2). Although many coin lesions are benign, some will turn out to be malignant. Despite the use of these strict criteria more than 50% of the coin lesions in their 124 patients were cancerous. Their review of 729 cases from the literature revealed a malignancy rate in coin lesions of approximately 37%. About 70% of their benign cases were granulomas. They concluded that, 'Exploratory thoracotomy is no longer a dangerous procedure [they operated on all 124 patients with no operative mortality]. It is recommended as a diagnostic procedure when other measures fail to provide a convincing defin-ition of a particular 'coin' lesion.' Today, fluoro-scopic or computerized tomographic guided percu-taneous biopsy is preferred to thoracotomy whenever possible.

'True coinage began soon after 650 BC. The sixth-century Greek poet Xenophanes, quoted by the historian Herodotus, ascribed its invention to the Lydians, 'the first to strike and use coins of gold and silver.'[3] The Peace dollar was the United States silver dollar from 1921–1935. It was the last silver dollar minted until the Eisenhower commemo-rative dollar was produced, beginning in 1971.

References
1. Ford, W.B., Kent, E.M., Neville, J.F. Jr and Fisher, D.L. (1956). 'Coin' lesions of the lung. *Am. Rev. Tuberc.*, 73, 134–8

2. Chiari, H.(1883). Zur kenntniss der Bronchialgeschwülste. *Prager Med. Wochenschr.*, 8, 497–9

3. Coins and coinage. In *The New Encyclopaedia Britannica*, 1990, 15th edn., Vol. 16, p. 531. (Chicago: Encyclopaedia Britannica Inc.)

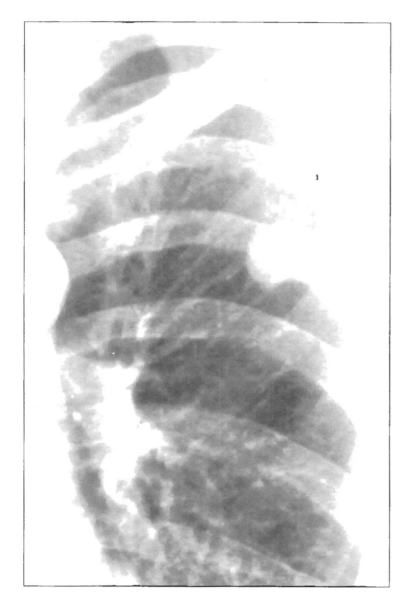

Figure 1. Chest radiograph showing solitary pulmonary nodule. Case courtesy of Dr C. White, University of Maryland

Figure 2. 1922 silver dollar (Peace dollar)

COOKIE BITE (COOKIE CUTTER) LESIONS

Metastatic lesions that are predominantly limited to the cortex of bone are unusual. They do, however, often produce a distinct pattern of destruction. This resembles bites along the edge of a cookie or the cutout in the dough left by a cookie cutter. Both of the terms (cookie bite and cookie cutter) are attributed to Andrew Deutsch and Donald Resnick (University of California and VA Medical Center, San Diego)[1]. They, along with Gen Niwayama, used the term cookie bites in the discussion of a 1981 case report of a patient with a bronchogenic carcinoma who had bone metastases.[2] They refer to an earlier paper 'submitted for publication' (their reference 2) with the term cookie bite in the title; however, that paper in its final published form[3] does not contain either term. Apparently the 'sign police' at the editorial office thwarted that attempt to embellish the literature with some picturesque language.

Publication histories aside, the recognition of metastatic disease is very important. Early recognition and treatment are helping to prolong a better quality of life for many cancer patients. Cortical 'cookie bite' lesions are seen most often with metastatic bronchogenic carcinomas (Figure 1). They can also be a manifestation of metastatic disease from several other cancers that metastasize to bone, especially breast carcinomas, renal cell carcinomas and thyroid cancers.

The word 'cookie' is derived from the 'Dutch koekje, diminutive of koek, 'cake'. [It refers to] any of various small sweet cakes, either flat or slightly raised, cut from rolled dough, dropped from a spoon, cut into pieces after baking, or curled with a special iron.'[4] Figure 2 shows a gingerbread man with cookie bite (leg) and cookie cutter (arm) 'lesions'.

References
1. Greenspan, A. and Norman, A. (1988). Osteolytic cortical destruction: an unusual pattern of skeletal metastases. *Skeletal Radiol.*, 17, 402–6

2. Deutsch, A., Resnick, D. and Niwayama, G. (1981). Case Report 145. *Skeletal Radiol.*, 6, 144–8

3. Deutsch, A. and Resnick, D. (1980). Eccentric cortical metastases to the skeleton from bronchogenic carcinoma. *Radiology,* 137, 49–52

4. Cookie. In *The New Encyclopaedia Britannica*, 1990, 15th edn., Vol. 3, p. 599. (Chicago: Encyclopaedia Britannica Inc.)

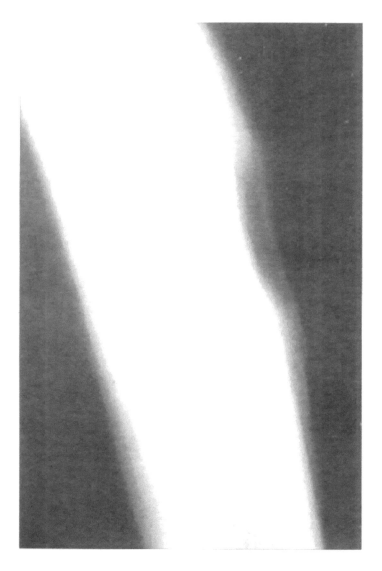

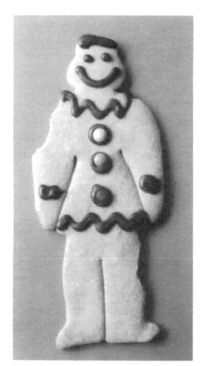

Figure 1. 'Focal area of cortical bone destruction involving the proximal femoral diaphysis.' Reprinted from Deutsch and Resnick[3]. Eccentric cortical metastases to the skeleton from bronchogenic carcinoma. *Radiology,* 1980;**137**, 49–52, with permission of the RSNA

Figure 2. Gingerbread man with cookie bite (leg) and cookie cutter (arm) 'lesions'

CORDUROY CLOTH VERTEBRA

Vertebral body hemangiomas have been described as striated or reticulated from the time of the earliest radiographic reports concerning these lesions. Rudolf Virchow (1821–1902) is credited with the first report (in 1862) of a vertebral hemangioma. 'The first publication in the English literature mentioning ... hemangioma goes back to the mid–nineteenth century [1845] when Toynbee[1] reported a single case involving the parietal bone'[2]. William Anspach[3] (Children's Memorial Hospital, Chicago) seems to have been the first to use the term corduroy cloth to describe the radiographic appearance. He wrote in 1937, 'An almost constant X-ray appearance has been produced, according to numerous recent reports, when hemangiomas involve vertebral bodies. Vertical streaks of parallel densities are seen on the roentgenograms somewhat resembling corduroy cloth. Older persons are especially prone to have this type of tumor. No other benign tumor has so uniformly produced these parallel densities.'[3] This sign is still considered characteristic (Figure 1). The parallel line appearance is due to reinforcement of the remaining vertical trabeculae within the vertebral body to make up for those lost because of the hemangioma. Occasionally, one may have difficulty distinguishing a Pagetoid vertebra from a vertebral hemangioma. Enlargement of the vertebral body associated with increased density is a clue that the changes are due to Paget's disease.

'Corduroy (Corde du Roi – woven for kings' servants in the Middle Ages) has extra wefts that form lengthwise rows of floats that are cut to form the pile [Figure 2]. This cloth was called thickset in the seventeenth and eighteenth centuries, and it is related to fustian, a sturdy wool or linen/cotton fabric dating back to the early centuries AD.'[4]

References

1. Toynbee, J. (1845). An account of two vascular tumors developed in the substance of bone. *Lancet* ii, 676

2. Huvos, A. G. (1979). *Bone Tumors*, p. 345. (Philadelphia: W. B. Saunders Co.)

3. Anspach, W.E. (1937). Sunray hemangioma of bone – with special reference to roentgen signs. *J. Am. Med. Assoc.*, 108, 617–20

4. Wilson, K. (1979). *A History of Textiles*, p. 69. (Boulder, CO: Westview Press)

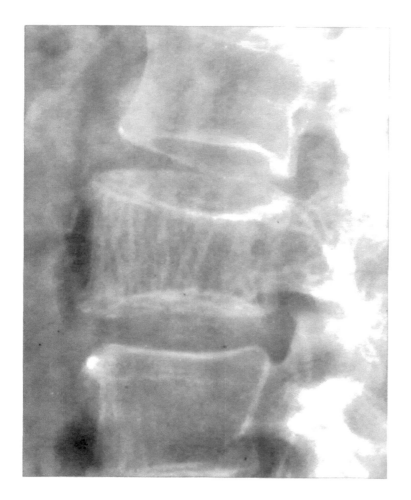

Figure 1. Lateral radiograph of spine showing vertical 'stripes' with a hemangioma (author's case)

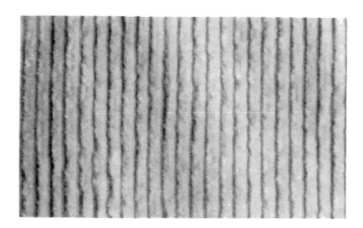

Figure 2. Corduroy cloth

COTTON WOOL SIGN

'It was [Vincenz] Czerny, in 1873, who first used the term 'osteitis deformans' to describe a condition of deformity and softening of the tibia and fibula in a young soldier. But it was not until 1876 that a clear account of the disease was rendered by Sir James Paget [1814–1899], who made a study of five cases.'[1]

Paget's disease affects the skeleton and results in several unusual appearances. One of these is the cotton wool pattern in the skull (Figure 1) (see also Picture frame, Blade of grass). Robert Roberts and Cohen[1] (Liverpool) used this term in their 1925 report of 16 cases of osteitis deformans. The skull X-ray of a 67-year-old man (their case II) showed 'small opaque areas are smaller and more numerous than in case I, and give an impression of multiple tufts of opaque cotton wool stuck to the surface of the skull.' In case XI, a 60-year-old man's skull X-ray outline was described as 'resembles that of the 'woolly head of a piccaninny'.' The simpler term, cotton wool, has endured. Today, the only other entity commonly considered in the differential diagnosis is osteoblastic metastatic disease.

'[A]rcheological evidence gives [cotton] a 'textile birth' sometime around 3500 BC in India ... Spun cotton yarns, dated at 3000 BC, were found in the ruins of Mohenjo-Daro, the great city in the Indus valley ... The cotton industry was well developed by 1500 BC'[2] (Figure 2).

'Mesopotamia was the 'land of wool' and the first place where sheep were domesticated. The tablets of Ur (2000 BC) tell of huge flocks of white and black sheep, of hundreds being shorn in a single day, of wool being sold and the prices received.'[2] Cotton wool is not a misnomer. It is a term used to describe raw cotton.

References
1. Roberts, R.E. and Cohen, M.J. (1925). Osteitis deformans (Paget's disease of bone). *Proc. R. Soc. Med.*, 19, 13–40

2. Wilson, K. (1979). *A History of Textiles*, pp. 16–24. (Boulder, CO: Westview Press)

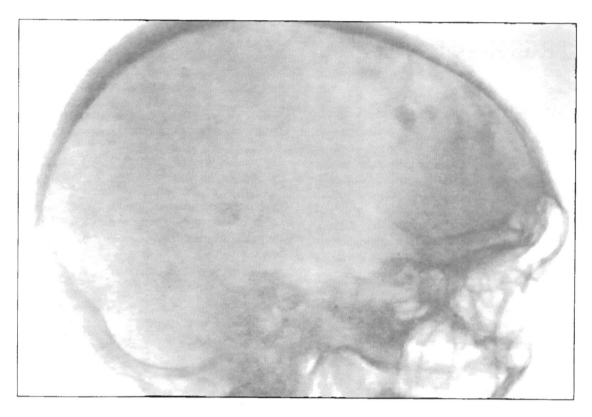

Figure 1. 'Paget's disease. Flattening. Inner table well
defined. Outer table thickened and ragged. Islands of dense
bone.' Reprinted from Roberts and Cohen[1]. Osteitis
deformans (Paget's disease of bone). *Proc. R. Soc. Med*, 1925,
19, 13–40, with permission of the Royal Society of Medicine

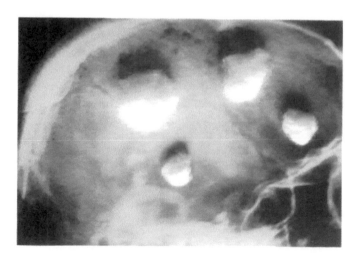

Figure 2. Cotton wool on skull X-ray

CRESCENT SIGN

A plain-film radiographic sign that would reliably indicate the presence of avascular necrosis at an early stage has eluded radiologists to date. Magnetic resonance imaging now gives us the ability to screen patients for this condition long before any plain-film signs are evident.

With their report of the crescent line in 1963, Alex Norman and Peter Bullough[1] thought that they had found that reliable early plain-film sign. It certainly is a classic indication of avascular necrosis. Further study of the natural history of avascular necrosis has shown, however, that this is not an early sign in the course of this disease. It is now considered a late sign that usually indicates impending collapse of the femoral head (Figure 1).

These two distinguished authorities at the Hospital for Joint Disease in New York City gave credit to three earlier authors for mentioning this finding before their work. Raymond Lewis[2] and Philip Jacobs[3] illustrated cases, with similar findings, in their discussions of Legg–Calve-Perthes' disease and osteochondritis dissecans of the hip, respectively. It was Jacobs[3] who stressed the importance of obtaining the 'frog leg' lateral view to detect subtle changes that were often not evident on the anteroposterior film. Henning Waldenström[4], in 1938, had observed a zone in the femoral head just underneath the position of the joint cartilage that he thought was 'caused by a subchondral resorption of necrotic bone.'

Norman and Bullough[1] in their pathologically proven study of '3 femoral heads removed from patients with avascular necrosis clearly establishe[d] the crescent-like zone of radiolucency as an area of subchondral separation [or fracture] and not resorption of necrotic bone.'

The *Oxford English Dictionary*[5] gives several definitions for the word crescent. The first is, 'The waxing moon, during the period between new moon and full.' Others include, 'The convexo-concave figure of the waxing or the waning moon, during the first or last quarter, especially when very new or very old' and 'A figure or outline of anything of this shape' (Figure 2).

The term, crescent sign, is also used to describe the appearance of obstructive hydronephrosis seen during excretory urography in infants and children. In this setting, it is known as the Dunbar crescent (said to have been first reported in 1959)[6].

References
1. Norman, A. and Bullough, P. (1963). The radiolucent crescent line – an early diagnostic sign of avascular necrosis of the femoral head. *Bull. Hosp. Joint Dis.*, 24, 99–104

2. Lewis, R.W. (1955). *The Joints of the Extremities*, p. 50. (Springfield, IL: Charles C. Thomas)

3. Jacobs, P. (1962). Osteochondritis dissecans of the hip. *Clin. Radiol.*, 13, 316–23

4. Waldenström, H. (1938). The first stages of coxa plana. *J. Bone Joint Surg.*, 20, 559–66

5. Simpson, J. and Weiner, E. (eds.) *Oxford English Dictionary*, 1989, 2nd edn, Vol. 4, p. 10. (Oxford: Clarendon Press)

6. Dunbar, J.S. and Nogrady, M.B. (1970). The calyceal crescent – a roentgenographic sign of obstructive hydronephrosis. *Am. J. Roentgenol.*, 110, 520–8

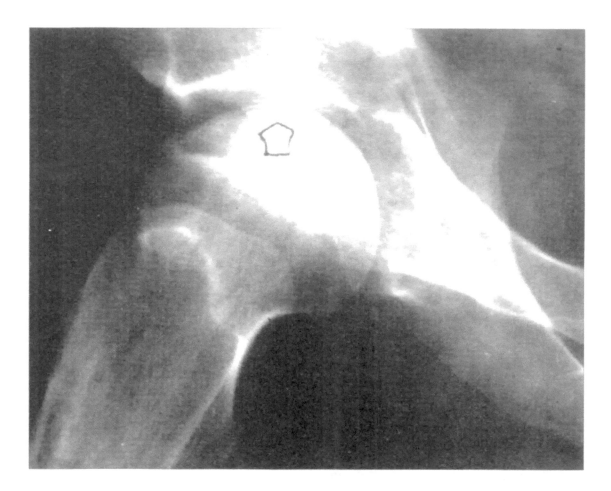

Figure 1. 'Arrow points to the Radiolucent Crescent Line.'
Reproduced from Norman and Bullough[1]. The radiolucent crescent
line – an early diagnostic sign of avascular nerosis of the femoral
head. *Bull. Hosp. Jovit Dis.,* **24**, 99–104, with permission from the
Bulletin of the Hospital for Joint Disease

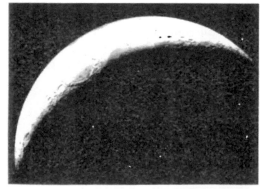

Figure 2. A crescent moon, from the
'Lick Observatory, 1937 September 9,
phase 4.16 days. Terminator at Rheita
Valley, Mare Foecunditatis, and Proclus.'
Lick Observatory photograph courtesy of
Lick Observatory, Mt Hamilton, CA

CUPID'S BOW VERTEBRA

Ted Keats[1] (University of Virginia, Charlottesville) has firmly established the importance of normal variant recognition for most radiologists in the United States with his books on normal roentgen variants. Alban Köhler and Emil-Alfred Zimmer did the same for generations of European radiologists with their classic 'Borderlands' text[2].

The term 'Cupid's bow' appeared in the literature in 1976[3]. It was introduced by Geral Dietz and Edward Christensen[3] (University of Texas, Southwestern) to describe a normal variation in the contour of the inferior end plates of the third, fourth and fifth lumbar vertebrae as seen on anteroposterior radiographs of the lumbar spine or abdomen (Figures 1 and 2). After initially noting this finding, they evaluated 200 lumbar spine studies and found the 'Cupid's bow' contour to some degree in 63.5% of the cases. They described the contour by stating, 'Rather than having a relatively flat inferior surface, the cortical margin of the inferior end plate in the frontal projection frequently simulates the curvature of a Cupid's bow aimed cephalad.'[3] It is important not to mistake this normal variant for some pathologic process that could cause bone weakness and deformity.

Cupid, son of Mercury and Venus, is the god of love in Roman mythology[4]. He shot arrows from his bow (Figure 3) to make the wounded gods or mortals fall hopelessly in love with whoever they happened to be gazing upon. Legend has it that his bow was carved from the club of Hercules.

References

1. Keats, T.E. (1995). *Atlas of Normal Roentgen Variants That May Simulate Disease*, 6th edn. (St Louis: Mosby-Year Book Inc.)

2. Schmidt, H. and Freyschmidt, J. (1993). *Köhler/Zimmer: Borderlands of Normal and Early Pathologic Findings in Skeletal Radiography*, 4th edn. (New York: Thieme Medical Publishers Inc.)

3. Dietz, G.W. and Christensen, E.E. (1976). Normal 'Cupid's Bow' contour of the lower lumbar vertebrae. *Radiology*, 121, 577–9

4. Tripp, E. (1970). *Crowell's Handbook of Classical Mythology*. (New York: Crowell)

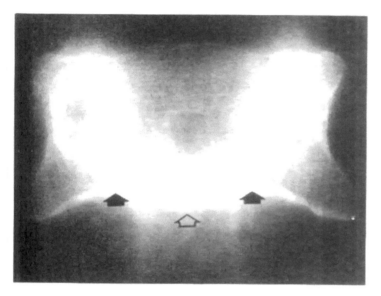

Figure 1. 'Anteroposterior tomogram of a lower lumbar vertebra reveals parasagittal concavities in the inferior end plate of the centrum. The contour simulates a Cupid's bow.'[1] Reprinted from Dietz and Christensen[3]. Normal 'Cupid's Bow' contour of the lower lumbar vertebrae. *Radiology*, 1976, **121**, 577–9, with permission of the RSNA

Figure 2. Radiograph of the lumbar spine demonstrates parasagittal concavities like those described by Dietz and Christensen[3] (author's case)

Figure 3. A cupid with his bow. Detail from Raphael's Galatea (1513) from Villa Farnesina, Rome

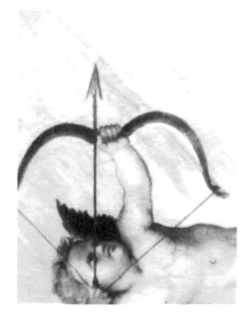

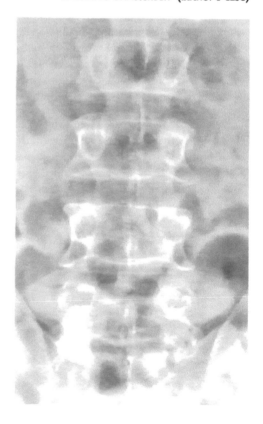

DELTA (EMPTY TRIANGLE) SIGN

Thrombotic occlusion of the cerebral venous sinuses is a disease entity with a high mortality rate. Within 5 years of the clinical introduction of computerized tomography (CT) scanners, Ferdinando Buonanno and his colleagues[1] (Bowman Gray School of Medicine) reported the CT findings of cerebral sinovenous occlusion in 11 patients with this disorder. Their paper appeared in the new *Journal of Computer Assisted Tomography* that is now known as *JCAT*. The overall mortality rate for their patients was 64%. They stressed the importance of accurate early diagnosis and found the 'delta' or 'empty triangle' sign to be pathognomonic for sagittal sinus thrombosis (Figure 1). The normal blood-filled triangular sinus is empty because there is a thrombus within its center. The empty triangle sign had to be seen 'on cuts at different levels to differentiate it from a high splitting of the SSS [superior sagittal sinus].' This sign can now also be detected with magnetic resonance imaging.

Delta is the fourth letter of the Greek alphabet (Figure 2). 'Most scholars are in agreement that the Greek alphabet is derived from the Phoenician [Semitic] and that it was developed between the 15th and 8th centuries BC, probably in the eleventh.'[2] In Hebrew, daleth is the name for the fourth letter of the north Semitic alphabet. The Hebrew word means 'door.' This is reportedly the origin of the Greek delta.

References

1. Buonanno, F.S., Moody, D.M., Ball, M.R. and Laster, D.W. (1978). Computed cranial tomographic findings in cerebral sinovenous occlusion. *J. Comput. Assist. Tomograph.*, 2, 281–90

2. Diringer, D. (1948). *The Alphabet – A Key to the History of Mankind*, pp. 218–452. (New York: Philosophical Library)

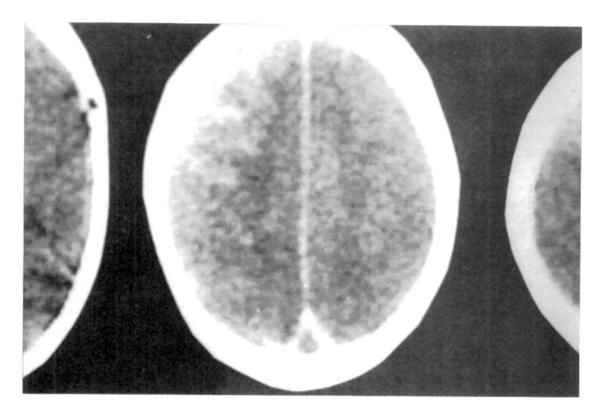

Figure 1. 'The 'empty triangle' or Δ sign – indicative of superior sagittal sinus thrombosis.' Reprinted from Buonanno et al.[1] Computed cranial tomographic findings in cerebral sinovenous occlusion. *J. Comput. Assist. Tomograph.*, 1978, **2**, 281–90, with permission of the author and Raven Press Ltd

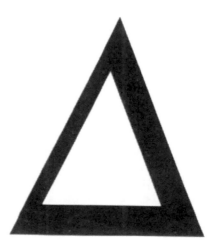

Figure 2. Greek letter delta

DOUGHNUT SIGN

Doughnut lesions in the brain, originally described on radioisotope brain scans, are now more familiar from their computerized tomography and magnetic resonance imaging appearances. 'Soon after the introduction of rectilinear scintillation scanning in 1955, focal organic lesions of the brain were delineated following the administration of various gamma-emitting compounds. Classically, these lesions have been identified as a locus of increased radioactivity within the low activity of normal brain tissue ... Since 1964, the use of large doses of short-lived agents, such as ^{99}mTc pertechnetate, has resulted in a better delineation of these lesions.'[1] This newer technology allowed Robert O'Mara and his colleagues[1], from the State University of New York in Syracuse, to note a pattern that differed from the classical one, i.e. a zone of increased uptake containing a central core of decreased activity – the doughnut sign (Figures 1 and 2). They studied more than 1400 scans in 18 months to determine the incidence and diagnostic significance of this sign. They credit Alexander Gottschalk and co-workers[2] for reporting a similar pattern. Their conclusion was that it 'is a relatively uncommon appearance since the pattern was observed in only 2.9 per cent of all positive studies [and was] of little value in indicating the etiology of a lesion.'[1] The doughnut sign had been seen in metastases, primary tumors, abscesses, hematomas and with cerebrovascular accidents. This still constitutes a significant list of differential diagnostic possibilities. 'The doughnut sign ... usually, though not invariably, indicates central necrosis, hemorrhage, or cyst formation within a lesion ... it may be helpful to the neurosurgeon to be forewarned that a lesion is likely to contain central necrosis or hemorrhage.'[1]

A doughnut is a 'small spongy cake made of dough (usually sweetened and spiced), and fried or boiled in lard. Frequently made in the shape of a thick ring'[3] (Figure 3).

The doughnut terminology (like the snack) is quite popular. It has also been used to describe abnormalities on cardiac radioisotope studies and for hilar adenopathy as seen on lateral chest radiographs.

References
1. O'Mara, R.E., McAfee, J.G. and Chodos, R.B. (1969). The 'doughnut' sign in cerebral radioisotopic images. *Radiology*, 92, 581–6

2. Gottschalk, A., Abatie, J.D., Petasnick, J.P., Polcyn, R.E., Beck, R.N. and Charleston, D.B. (1968). The comparison between sensitivity and resolution based on a clinical evaluation with the ACRH brain scanner. Presented at the *IAEA Symposium on Medical Radioisotope Scintigraphy*, Salzburg, Austria, August

3. Doughnut. In Simpson, J. and Weiner, E. (eds.) *Oxford English Dictionary*, 1989, 2nd edn., Vol. 4, p. 987. (Oxford: Clarendon Press)

Figure 1. 'Anterior scan demonstrates a large area of increased radioactivity surrounding a central area of decreased activity. This is consistent with the 'doughnut sign' of central necrosis.' Reprinted from O'Mara et al.[1] The doughnut sign in cerebral radioisotopic images. *Radiology,* 1969, **92,** 581–6, with permission of the RSNA

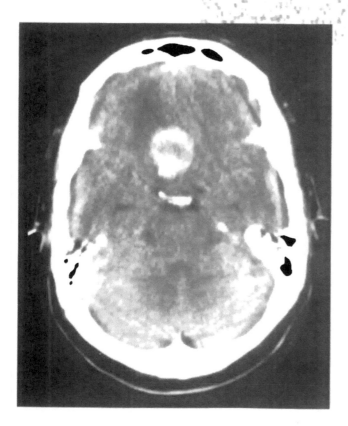

Figure 2. Computerized tomograph of the head of a patient with bleeding aneurysm showing doughnut pattern with hyperdense periphery and central area of decreased attenuation. Case courtesy of Dr M. Rothman, University of Maryland

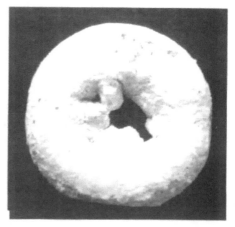

Figure 3. A sugar doughnut

DRIPPING CANDLEWAX SIGN

One of the few radiologic signs imparting a sense of motion to our two-dimensional static images is the description of melorheostosis as dripping candlewax ('en coulée'). This term was used by André Léri and Joanny[1] when they reported this condition for the first time in 1922 at the Medical Society of Paris Hospitals. They also proposed the term, melorheostosis, for the name of the new disorder. Their patient was then a 39-year-old woman who had noticed deformities of her left index and long fingers since the age of 10. She later developed difficulty with her left elbow and shoulder. On X-ray examination performed at that time, 'it seemed as if an opaque mass had been dripped all along the bones of the limb.' The edges of the hyperostosis are most often very bumpy – comparable to the surface of dripping candlewax. The appearance is characteristic (Figure 1). There is usually no need to list a differential diagnosis. Léri and Joanny did not speculate on the pathogenesis or etiology of this disorder. The cause and pathogenesis are still unknown.

'The true candle probably arrived in the days of the Romans ... Pliny, in the first century AD, refers to Greek and Roman candles of flax threads coated with pitch and wax ... During the Middle Ages and right up to the early days of the nineteenth century, the commoner candles were made of tallow ... The first departure from the centuries-old alternatives of tallow and beeswax came with the opening up of the sperm-whale fishery in the eighteenth century. Spermaceti came into use for candle-making near the end of that century. Spermaceti candles became, and are still used as, a standard measure of artificial light; the term so often used, one 'candle-power', being based on the light given by a pure spermaceti candle.'[2] (Figure 2).

References

1. Léri, A. and Joanny (1922). Une affection non décrite des os: hyperostose 'en coulée' sur toute la longueur d'un membre ou 'mélorhéostose.' *Bull. Mem. Soc. Méd. Hóp. Paris*, 46, 1141–5

2. Robins, F.W. (1970). *The Story of the Lamp (and the Candle)*, pp. 16–20. (Bath: Kingsmead Reprints)

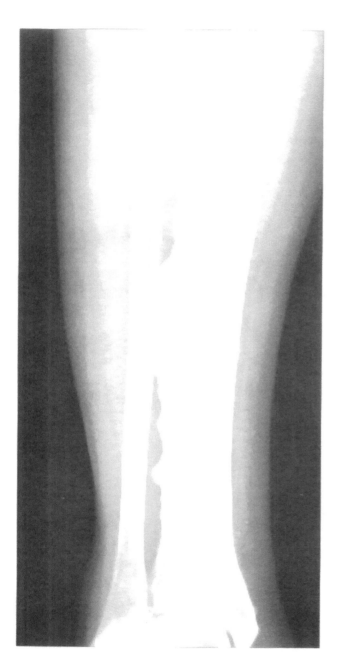

Figure 1. Radiograph showing typical 'flowing' bone formation along cortex of tibia. Case courtesy of Dr C. Resnik, University of Maryland

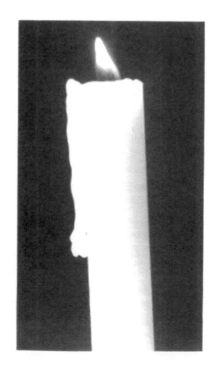

Figure 2. A burning candle with dripping wax

DROMEDARY KIDNEY

A dromedary or humped kidney, is a normal variant contour of the left kidney seen in about 2% of patients (Figure 1); it is rarely seen on the right kidney. 'An appropriate designation for this morphology would be the term, dromedary left kidney.'[1] This term and the normal variant it describes was discussed in a 1962 report from the University of Miami and Mercy Hospital, by Benedict Harrow and Jack Sloane[1]. They studied 1000 consecutive excretory urograms in adults, noting the 'peculiarity' in 23 patients. They had recognized the humped kidney for several years but stated it was 'not until nephrography became more routine during intravenous urography [that] this entity [could] be more clearly defined.' They acknowledged Johan Frimann-Dahl's 1961 paper[2] as the only other publication to address this deformity. He reported a 10% prevalence in nearly 6000 cases and attributed the contour deformity to prolonged splenic pressure on the renal surface. Harrow and Sloane[1] found no relationship with the splenic shadow. The dromedary hump should simply be recognized as a normal variant and not mistaken for a renal mass lesion. (See Beak sign.)

'The extant Camelidae are classed in two genera. The Old World genus of *Camelus* is generally accepted to comprise two species: *C. dromedarius*, the dromedary, one-humped or Arabian camel [Figure 2]; and *C. bactrianus*, the Bactrian or two-humped camel ... In the new world there also exists a single genus of the Camelidae, comprising four species'[3] including the guanaco, vicuña, llama and alpaca. 'Like the horse, the camel has its origins in North America.'[3] Its ancestors, the Tylopoda, were recognizable 50 million years ago.

References

1. Harrow, B.R. and Sloane, J.A. (1962). The dromedary or humped left kidney. *Am. J. Roentgenol.*, 88, 144–52

2. Frimann-Dahl, J. (1961). Normal variations of the left kidney. *Acta Radiol.*, 55, 207–16

3. Wilson, R.T. (1984). *The Camel*, pp. 1–2. (London: Longman Group Ltd)

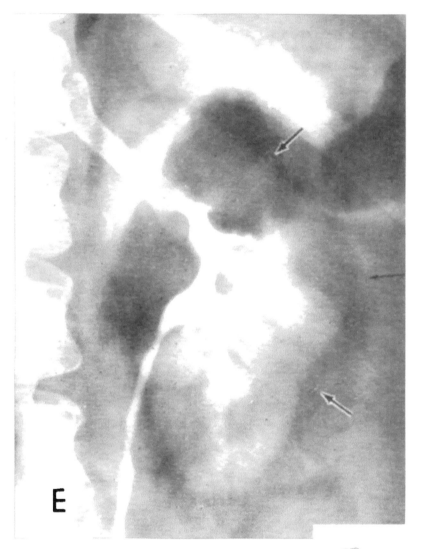

E

Figure 1. 'Arrows point to the humped portion of a typical triangular-shaped left kidney visualized during intravenous urography.' Reprinted from Harrow and Sloane[1]. The dromedary or humped left kidney. *Am. J. Roentgenol.*, 1962, **88**, 144–52, with permission of the ARRS

Figure 2. 'Camels in the Kalahari desert.' Reprinted from Wilson[3]. *The Camel.* London: Longman Group Ltd 1984. Photograph from Barnaby's Picture Library with permission

EGG SHAPED (EGG-ON-A-STRING) HEART

The first description of the characteristic configuration of the heart in young patients with complete transposition of the great vessels is said to have been done by Helen Taussig[1] in 1938. Many years later (1964) the term 'egg-shaped' was used in a report by Lewis Carey and Larry Elliott[2] to describe this characteristic configuration. (Elliott had coined the phrase, personal communication). They reported a series of 47 patients with complete transposition and studied both the radiographs and necropsy specimens. 'In the frontal projection, the configuration of the heart was usually quite characteristic: it was similar to the shape of an egg, tilted so that its long axis lay in an oblique direction. The pole with the least convexity lay upwards and to the right; the pole with the greatest convexity lay downwards and to the left'[2] (Figure 1). Recognizing the abnormal shape of the heart is one of the key elements that will allow for a correct diagnosis in congenital heart disease cases. Other important factors include: position of the aortic knob, size of the main pulmonary artery, evaluation of the pulmonary vascularity and determination of visceral situs.

Modification of the egg (Figure 2) was an important step in the evolution of reptiles. 'The two innovations ... perhaps most crucial in effecting the transition from the amphibian to the reptilian state were the cornification of the skin and the protection of the embryo by membranes and a shell'[3] (i.e. an eggshell). The first reptiles (captorhinomorphs) appeared in the mid-Carboniferous times, about 320 million years ago. The oldest egg in paleontologists' possession was found in the Texas red beds formed during the early part of the Permian period, about 280 million years ago.

References
1. Nogrady, M.B. and Dunbar, J.S. (1969). Complete transposition of the great vessels. *J. Can. Assoc. Radiol.*, 20, 124–31

2. Carey, L.S. and Elliott, L.P. (1964). Complete transposition of the great vessels. *Am. J. Roentgenol.*, 91, 529–43

3. Stahl, B.J. (1974). *Vertebrate History: Problems in Evolution*, pp. 251–9. (New York: McGraw-Hill Inc.)

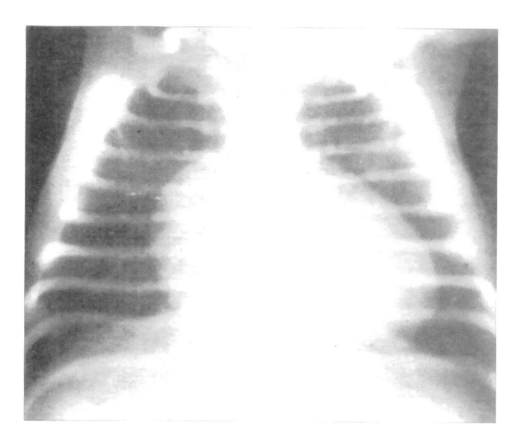

Figure 1. Egg-shaped heart due to 'complete transposition of the great vessels with intact ventricular septum (male, aged 2 days; 1.5 mm patent ductus).' Reprinted from Carey and Elliott[2]. Complete transposition of the great vessels. *Am. J. Roentgenol.*, 1964, **91**, 529–43, with the permission of the ARRS

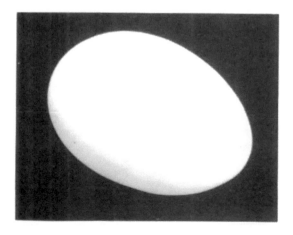

Figure 2. Grade A large egg

EGG-SHELL CALCIFICATIONS

Allen Riemer's 1945 article[1], from the Denver Municipal Tuberculosis Dispensary, on 'Egg-shell calcifications in silicosis', attributes the origin of the term egg-shell to Henry Sweany and colleagues[2] (Chicago Municipal Tuberculosis Sanitarium) who used it in their article 'Chemical and Pathologic Study of Pneumoconiosis.'[2] The roentgen findings from this work, including a discussion of 'egg-shell' calcification, were reported separately by Sweany in an article[3] that appeared in print 5 months before the major paper. Although this predates the main paper[2], the main paper was presented before either publication at the Annual Session of the American Medical Association in Kansas City, Missouri on May 13th, 1936. It is the main chemical and pathologic paper, not the radiographic article, that contains a photo showing the 'egg-shell' type calcifications seen in a specimen roentgenogram of some hilar lymph nodes from a patient with borderline silicosis and silicotuberculosis (Figure 1).

Publication dates aside, Sweany and colleagues[2] reported a detailed analysis of 40 patients with pneumoconiosis and found an infiltration of calcium underneath the capsule of lymph nodes (Figure 2). This led them to use the term 'egg-shell' (Figure 3) calcification. This was noted in silicosis patients who had tuberculosis as an additional complication. The calcification was felt to be caused by the tuberculosis.

Later investigators have shown that uncomplicated cases of silicosis may also have 'egg-shell' calcifications. Today, this is the entity classically thought of in association with the finding. Irradiated nodes in lymphoma patients may also show this type of calcification.

(See Egg shaped sign for a discussion of the egg shell.)

References
1. Riemer, A.D. (1945). Egg-shell calcification in silicosis. *Am. J. Roentgenol.*, 53, 439–45
2. Sweany, H.C., Porsche, J.D. and Douglass, J.R. (1936). Chemical and pathologic study of pneumoconiosis. *Arch. Pathol.*, 22, 593–633
3. Sweany, H.C. (1936). Pathologic interpretations of roentgenologic shadows in pneumoconiosis. *J. Am. Med. Assoc.*, 106, 1959–65

Figure 1. 'A roentgenogram of the hilar lymph nodes in case 11, revealing calcification of the 'egg-shell' type.' Reprinted from Sweany *et al.*[2] Chemical and pathologic study of pneumoconiosis. *Arch. Pathol.*, 1936, **22**, 593–633. Copyright 1936, American Medical Association

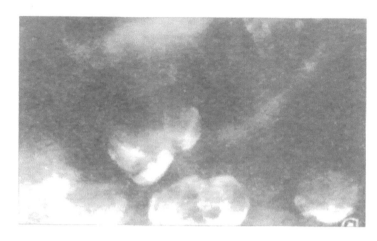

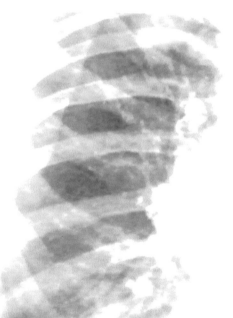

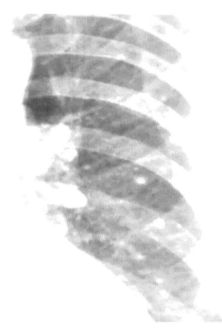

Figure 2. Chest radiograph of patient with egg-shell calcification of hilar lymph nodes. Case courtesy of Dr C. White, University of Maryland

Figure 3. Shell from grade A large egg

ERLENMEYER FLASK DEFORMITY

Philippe Gaucher[1] described the condition that now bears his name in 1882. This cerebroside disorder leads to packing of the bone marrow with lipid-laden reticuloendothelial cells and causes modeling abnormalities that are especially well demonstrated in the metaphyses of the long bones. The earliest detailed descriptions of the clinical, radiologic and pathologic findings were presented in two separate articles[2,3], from the same case material, in 1926. The radiologist involved, Sven Junghagen (Röntgeninstitut Lund), described the abnormal contour of the ends of the long bones in a 3-year-old girl who had clinical and radiographic follow up over a 2-year period. However, it was A.W. Fisher (University of Frankfurt) who seems to have first used the term flask-shaped (flaschenförmige) in an article 2 years later[4] (Figure 1). He discussed the long bone changes, especially those in the distal femur, in 16 cases. Nine of the patients had a diagnosis of Gaucher's disease. The others had diagnoses that included: Pick's disease, chronic osteomyelitis, arthritis deformans and pernicious anemia. Fisher emphasized that the differences and similarities between cases, that may occur in the shape of the distal femur, are dependent upon the specific disease process involved. Thus, this Erlenmeyer flask-shaped deformity is not specific for Gaucher's disease. It can be seen with many other disorders especially marrow-packing disorders. The long bone radiographic changes in what is now known as Niemann–Pick's disease are indistinguishable from those due to Gaucher's disease.

The laboratory flask commonly used in Fisher's time, as it still is today, was that invented by Richard Erlenmeyer in 1861 (Figure 2). He was a professor of chemistry at Munich Polytechnic School. He is also remembered, by chemists, for synthesizing several important organic compounds[5].

References

1. Gaucher, P. (1882). De l'epithélioma primitif de la rate; hypertrophie idiopathique de la rate sans leucémie. *Thèse*, Paris

2. Junghagen, S. (1926). Röntgenologische Skelettveränderungen bei Morbus Gaucher. *Acta Radiol.*, 5, 506–15

3. Klercker, O. (1926–7). Beiträge zur Kenntnis des Morbus Gaucher, besonders in klinischer Hinsicht. *Acta Paediatr.*, 6, 302–51

4. Fisher, A.W. (1928). Das Röntgenbild der Knochen, besonders des Femur in der Diagnose des Morbus Gaucher. *Fortschr. Geb. Röntgenstr.*, 37, 158–64

5. *Academic American Encyclopedia*, 1982, Vol. 7, p. 231. (Danbury, CT: Grolier Inc.)

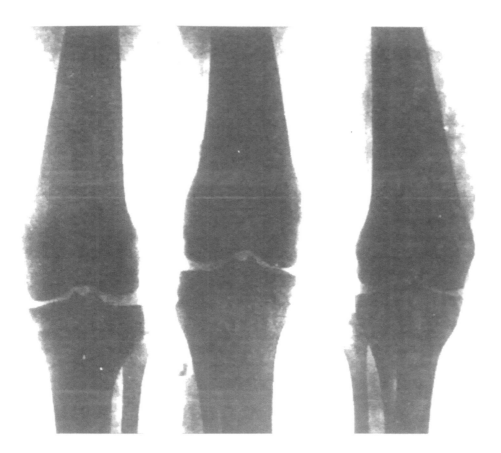

Figure 1. Erlenmeyer flask-shaped deformity shown in radiographs of patients with Gaucher's disease and deformity of the distal femur. Reproduced from Fisher[4]. Das Röntgenbild der Knochen, besonders des Femur in der Diagnose des Morbus Gaucher. *Fortschr. Geb. Rontgenstr.*, 1928, **37**, 158–64, with permission

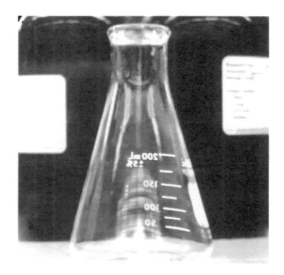

Figure 2. An Erlenmeyer flask

FOOTBALL SIGN

Roscoe Miller[1], one of America's great gastro-intestinal radiologists, gave a presentation on this 'new' sign at the forty-fifth meeting of the Radiological Society of North America that was held in Chicago, Illinois, 15–20 November 1959. The 'football' or 'air-dome' sign was reported to be pathognomonic of pneumoperitoneum. A large oval air collection, within the abdomen, was divided superiorly by the vertical streak of the falciform ligament (Figure 1). Its recognition in newborns and infants as a sign of a perforated viscus was emphasized, since spontaneous non-traumatic rupture of the intestinal tract in infants was an unusual condition with a grave prognosis. The first diagnosis of pneumoperitoneum in the United States is said to have occurred in March 1918. William N. Beggs and William W. Wasson made the diagnosis of pneumoperitoneum after trying to induce a therapeutic pneumothorax[2].

Miller was on the staff at Indiana University, at the time of his report, and is said to have been a fan of the school's football team (Henry Wellman, personal communication). These were the days of Johnny Unitas, Jimmy Brown, Paul Hornung, Pat Summerall, Y.A. Tittle, Frank Gifford, Vince Lombardi and George Halas. The Baltimore Colts were the defending champions. They had beaten the New York Giants in New York 23–17 in sudden death overtime to win the 1958 cham-pionship game and they were destined to become champions again in 1959 when they would beat the Giants again 31–16[3].

American football developed from British rugby. A plaque in the lobby of the gymnasium at Rutgers University in New Jersey informs the football pilgrim that 'Here, November 6, 1869 took place the First Intercollegiate Football Contest ever held.' Their opponents were the Princeton University Tigers; Rutgers won 6–4. This game was more like rugby than football as we know it. There were 15 men on each side and there was no 'line of scrimmage'. The credit for the modifica-tions that made the game more like that played today goes to Walter Chauncey Camp (1859–1925). Brought up in New Haven, Connecticut, Walter entered Yale University in 1876. He played halfback and captained the team in 1878 and 1879. He proposed the changes to the governing association in 1880 that allowed the teams undisputed possession of the ball in the scrimmage and that reduced the number of players from 15 to 11[4]. In 1934 the ball (Figure 2) was changed to a shape (prolate spheroid) that was better for passing[5].

References

1. Miller, R.E. (1960). Perforated viscus in infants: a new roentgen sign. *Radiology*, 74, 65–7

2. Grigg, E.R.N. (1965). *The Trail of the Invisible Light*, p. 862. (Springfield, IL: Charles C. Thomas)

3. Neft, D.S. and Cohen, R.M. (1991). *The Football Encyclopedia. The Complete History of Professional NFL Football from 1892 to the Present*, pp. 272–9. (New York: St. Martin's Press)

4. Weyand, A.M. (1955). *The Saga of American Football*, pp. 1–21. (New York: Macmillan Company)

5. Hickok, R. (1992). *The Encyclopedia of North American Sports History*, p. 164. (New York: Facts on File)

Figure 1. The football sign seen in a 'three-day-old male with normal forty-week gestation. Although there is slight rotation, the large oval divided superiorly by the streak of the falciform ligament is easily seen.' Reprinted from Miller[1]. Perforated viscus in infants. *Radiology*, 1960, **74**, 65–7, with permission of the RSNA

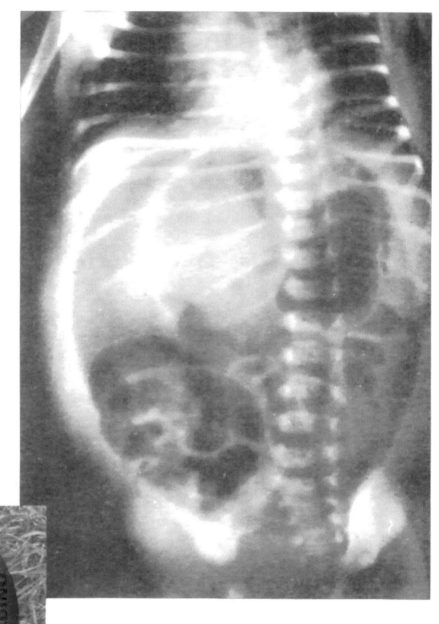

Figure 2. An American football

GREENSTICK FRACTURE

Joseph Malgaigne[1] (1806–1865) tells us that the first reference to incomplete fractures or curvatures of bone is Glazer's 1673 autopsy report of a 12-year-old boy with such an injury in the femur. 'A child, twelve years old, in jumping, felt pain in his thigh. He could, for two days, walk and go down stairs, putting the point of the foot to the ground; after which there ensued an acute inflammation, and a copious suppuration, which carried him off.'[1]

Daniel Turner[2] (1667–1741) (College of Physicians, London) in his 1722 writings on incomplete fractures said, 'when by some Force or Violence externally offer'd to one Side, the same gives way by bending, but the Bony Fibres on the opposite being thus hard press'd, and not capable to hold longer upon the like Flexion, snap asunder, after the Manner of a Stick, not over dry [i.e. a greenstick], bent to such a Degree as to strain the ligneous Fibres, and put them, tho whole on their Concave, upon flying asunder on their Convexity, and splitting perhaps half way through [Figure 1]. These Accidents usually attend Children and Infants, whose Bony Stria and Lamina are more ductile and pliable than in the Adult.'[2]

Turner's observations still hold true. Greenstick and buckle or torus fractures are most commonly seen today in the distal radius and ulna of children 5–10 years old. The greenstick fracture, as described by Turner, is due to a bending force applied perpendicular to the shaft of a long bone, just like the force applied to a stick broken over the knee (Figure 2). A buckle or torus fracture occurs when the force is transmitted along (parallel to) the long axis of the shaft. The latter is commonly seen after a fall on the outstretched hand (FOOSH).

'After the initial invasion of land by plants, perhaps 500 million years ago, the evolution of the first trees [and their green sticks] began; not until the Devonian Period (345 million to 395 million years ago) did the first vascular plants, including some treelike forms, appear. The Devonian was succeeded by the Carboniferous Period (280 million to 345 million years ago), during which the climate of most of the world was uniformly warm and moist. It favoured the growth of trees, and numerous kinds, many of gigantic size, evolved and populated the vast forests characteristic of that period.'[3]

References

1. Malgaigne, J.F. (1859). *A Treatise on Fractures*, translated by Packard, J.H., p. 50. (Philadelphia: J.B. Lippincott)

2. Turner, D. (1722). Of fractures incompleat. In *The Art of Surgery*, Vol. 2, pp. 169–71. (London: C. Rivington)

3. Trees. In *The New Encyclopaedia Britannica*, 1990, 15th edn, Vol. 8, pp. 879–83. (Chicago: Encyclopaedia Britannica Inc.)

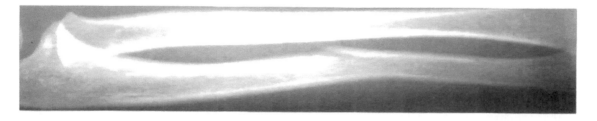

Figure 1. Greenstick fracture seen in a lateral radiograph of forearm showing incomplete fracture of the ulna (author's case)

Figure 2. A broken green stick

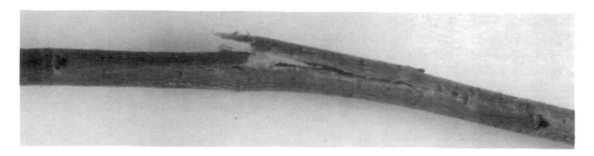

GROUND GLASS PATTERN

'Fibrous dysplasia of the bone, a pathologic entity of the bone characterized by extensive proliferation of fibrous tissue, which destroys and replaces normal bone elements, was differentiated from generalized fibrocystic disease of the bone caused by hyperfunction of the parathyroid glands by Hunter, et al.'[1,2] in 1931. The classic clinical, pathologic and roentgenographic appearance was described by Louis Lichtenstein[3] (Hospital for Joint Disease, New York) in 1938. He reported eight cases of polyostotic fibrous dysplasia drawn to his attention by Henry Jaffe. The first case report in the article concerns a 19-year-old woman whose right femur roentgenograms showed 'broadening and rarefaction of the upper two thirds. The cortex of the bone was thin ... the osseous structure had a hazy, ground glass, trabeculated appearance'[3] (Figure 1). A follow-up article by Lichtenstein and Jaffe[4] further explained the radiographic findings by stating, 'The rarefactions reflect the replacement, in the affected area, of the spongy bone and of the adjacent inner surface of the cortex by fibrous connective tissue, which, of course, is relatively radiolucent. If within this tissue there has been substantial metaplastic ossification, the rarefaction shadow is likely to present a mottled or rather cloudy ground glass appearance.'[4] Recognition of a bone tumor's matrix mineralization pattern (fibrous, chondroid or osseous) is one of the key factors involved in making a specific diagnosis. The ground glass pattern is indicative of a fibrous tissue matrix (Figures 2 and 3).

'When and where glass was invented will remain a mystery, as is the case with most of the primitive technical achievements of prehistoric man ... [B]eads and amulets of coloured glass were known to the Egyptians in the fourth millenium BC.'[5] 'One of the very early glass recipes ... was written in Mesopotamia on a clay tablet in a cuneiform script that is dated between the fourteenth and twelfth centuries BC.'[6]

Ground glass is also a term for abnormalities of the lung seen with high resolution computerized tomography scanning.

References

1. Firat, D. and Stutzman, L. (1968). Fibrous dysplasia of the bone. Am. J. Med., 44, 421–9

2. Hunter, D. and Turnbull, H.M. (1931). Hyperparathyroidism: generalized osteitis fibrosa. Br. J. Surg., 19, 203–84

3. Lichtenstein, L. (1938). Polyostotic fibrous dysplasia. Arch. Surg., 36, 874–98

4. Lichtenstein, L. and Jaffe, H.L. (1942). Fibrous dysplasia of bone. Arch. Pathol., 33, 777–816

5. Neuburg, F. (1962). Ancient Glass, p. 1. (Toronto: University of Toronto Press)

6. Tait, H. (1991). Glass – 5000 years, p. 8. (New York: Harry N. Abrams Inc.)

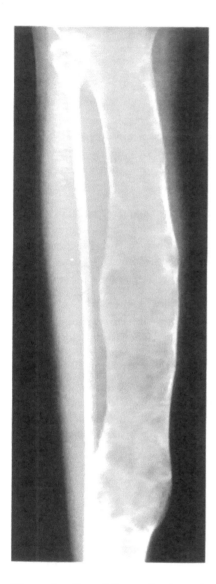

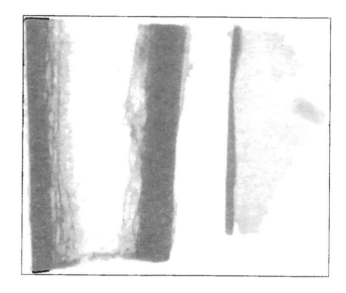

Figure 1. 'Roentgenogram of a portion of a diseased tibia [on right], illustrating the marked thinning of the cortex, the absence of deposition of periosteal bone, the endosteal erosion of the cortex and the filling of the medullary cavity by a homogeneous fibrous tissue containing tiny spicules of bone. Compare with the normal tibia on the left.' Reprinted from Lichtenstein[3]. Polyostotic fibrous dysplasia. *Arch. Surg.*, 1938, **36**, 874–98. Copyright 1938, American Medical Association

Figure 2. Typical fibrous dysplasia of the tibia (author's case)

Figure 3. Photograph (A) and radiograph (B) of tibia. Medullary space filled with ground glass. Ground glass courtesy of Sylvio and Jean Bettio, Chipped Glass and Crystal Repair Service, Clifton, NJ. Specimen radiograph by Jay Meyers, Registered Radiologic Technologist (RRT)

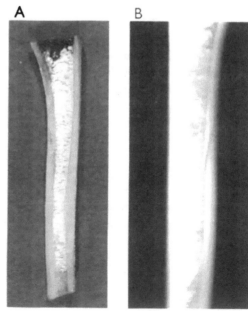

GULL WINGS AND MOUSE EARS

The recognition of the various patterns of arthritic destruction and the specific target areas involved, in each arthritic disorder, are the key factors used by the radiologist to make the correct diagnosis. The 1980 paper by William Martel and colleagues[1] discussed the specific patterns of destruction that differentiate psoriatic arthritis (PA) from erosive osteoarthritis (EOA). Martel and his colleagues, at the University of Michigan, reported the findings in 84 patients who had either psoriatic arthritis or erosive osteoarthritis. The erosions on the distal surface of the distal interphalangeal joints (in patients with PA) have a characteristic appearance which suggests 'mouse ears' (Figure 1).

A gull-wing deformity of a phalanx in the hand (especially the distal phalanx) may result from the erosive pattern seen in patients with erosive osteoarthritis (Figure 2). Central erosions in the distal ends of the middle phalanges are the key findings that allow a diagnosis of EOA to be made. Martel and his colleagues[1] said, 'The erosions of the [interphalangeal] joints in EOA are largely a consequence of destruction of the articular cartilage. The resultant deformity of the distal subchondral cortex suggests 'gull wings' because the most marked bone erosion is peripheral, whereas on the proximal side of the joint, the erosion is usually most marked near the center of the bone.'[1] The disease process was first described by Darrell Crain[2] (Georgetown University) in 1961. The term 'erosive osteoarthritis' first appeared in two 1966 articles by J.B. Peter and colleagues[3,4]. In my opinion a similar deformity, without erosions, is seen at the base of the distal phalanges in patients with advanced simple 'degenerative' osteoarthritis.

Anne Brower refers to this pattern of erosive change as the seagull deformity (personal communication). Martel says that he had no particular bird in mind at the time (personal communication).

Gulls are widely-ranging essentially marine birds classified in the Order Charadriiform, family *Laridae* (Figure 3). They are always inclined to be gregarious. Perhaps the most famous seagull is Jonathan Livingston Seagull whose story was widely read in the 1970s[5].

The mouse whose rounded ears are most like the rounded erosions seen in patients with psoriatic arthritis might be Mickey Mouse or one of his compatriots (Figure 4). Mickey's history is given in the discussion of the Mickey Mouse Sign. Martel says that he had no particular mouse in mind at the time the term was coined, although he does agree that Mickey's ears would make suitable models (personal communication).

References

1. Martel, W., Stuck, K.J., Dworin, A.M. and Hylland, R.G. (1980). Erosive osteoarthritis and psoriatic arthritis: a radiologic comparison in the hand, wrist and foot. *Am. J. Roentgenol.*, 134, 125–35

2. Crain, D.C. (1961). Interphalangeal osteoarthritis. *J. Am. Med. Assoc.*, 175, 1049–53

3. Kidd, K.L. and Peter, J.B. (1966). Erosive osteoarthritis. *Radiology,* 86, 640–7

4. Peter, J.B., Pearson, C.M. and Marmor, L. (1966). Erosive osteoarthritis of the hands. *Arthritis Rheum.*, 9, 365–88

5. Bach, R. (1970). *Jonathan Livingston Seagull.* (New York: Avon Books)

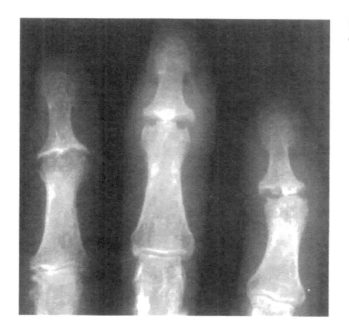

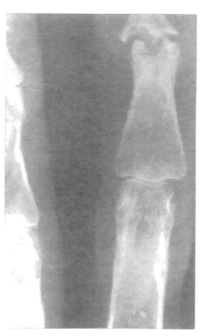

Figure 1. Radiograph showing erosions of psoriatic arthritis ('mouse ears')

Figure 2. 'Erosive osteoarthritis. Typical subchondral erosions of DIP [distal interphalangeal] joints causing 'gull wings' configuration.' Reprinted from Martel et al.[1]. Erosive osteoarthritis and psoriatic arthritis: a radiologic comparison in the hand, wrist and foot. *Am. J. Roentgenol.*, 1980, **134**, 125–35

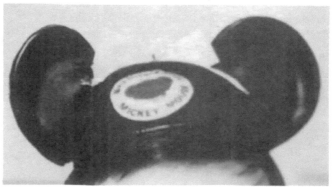

Figure 4. Mouse-ear memorabilia

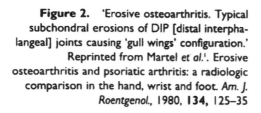

Figure 3. A seagull in flight.

HAIR-ON-END PATTERN

Sickle cell anemia was described by James B. Herrick[1] (1861–1954) in 1910, after his intern (Ernest E. Irons) saw and recorded peculiarly-shaped red blood corpuscles in a 20-year-old Grenadian dental student who was seen as a patient at Presbyterian Hospital, Chicago, in 1904. This patient was attended by Irons and Herrick until he (the patient) graduated from the Chicago College of Dental Surgery and returned to Grenada[2].

Sickle cell disease is rarely mentioned in the medical literature again until the late 1920s. The skull X-ray findings, first described by Thomas Cooley and Pearl Lee[3] in 1925, were, until 1936, described by them and other authors[4] as vertical or radiating lines. Cassie Rose[5] used the phrase, projecting 'like a porcupine's quills.' However, in the 1937 report by Lemuel Diggs and colleagues[6] (University of Tennessee) one finds a skull X-ray with the term 'hair-on-end' trabeculations (Figure 1). This term is now classically associated with the skull radiographic changes seen in sickle cell disease and even more classically with the changes due to Cooley's anemia (thalassemia major).

The 'hair' represents the accentuated trabeculae extending between the inner and outer skull tables in the expanded diploic marrow space. This 'hair' appears to be 'on end' because these fine strand-like trabeculae are orientated perpendicular to the skull's inner and outer tables.

Hair is one of the characteristics that distinguishes the zoologic class Mammalia from other classes of earthly creatures (Figure 2).

References

1. Herrick, J.B. (1910). Peculiar elongated and sickle-shaped red blood corpuscles in a case of severe anemia. *Arch. Intern. Med.*, 6, 517–21

2. Savitt, T.L. and Goldberg, M.F (1989). Herrick's 1910 case report of sickle cell anemia. *J. Am. Med. Assoc.*, 261, 266–71

3. Cooley, T.B. and Lee, P. (1925). A series of cases of anemia with splenomegaly and peculiar bone changes. *Trans. Am. Pediatr. Soc.*, 37, 29

4. LeWald, L.T. (1932). Roentgen evidence of osseous manifestations in sickle-cell (drepanocytic) anemia and in mediterranean (erythroblastic) anemia. *Radiology*, 18, 792–8

5. Rose, C.B. (1929). Some unusual X-ray findings in skulls. *Radiology*, 13, 508–14

6. Diggs, L.W., Pulliam, H.N. and King, J.C. (1937). The bone changes in sickle cell anemia. *South. Med. J.*, 30, 249–59

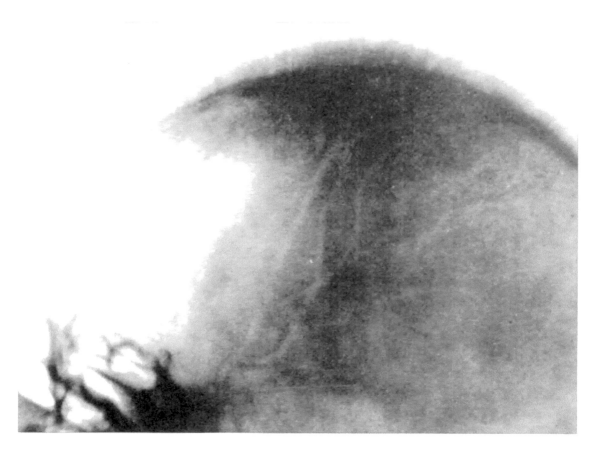

Figure 1. 'Sickle cell anemia. Osteoporosis of vertex, diploic widening, absence of distinct outer table, hair-on-end trabeculations.'[6] Reprinted from Diggs et al.[6] The bone changes in sickle cell anemia. *South. Med. J.,* 1937, **30,** 249–59, with permission

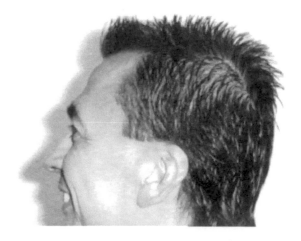

Figure 2. Hair-on-end style haircut

HITCH-HIKER'S THUMB

One of the characteristic findings in patients with diastrophic dwarfism (diastrophic dysplasia) is hypoplasia of the first metacarpal. This metacarpal hypoplasia results in a low-set, laterally directed thumb, the hitch-hiker's thumb. Although this abnormality was emphasized in the 1960 article[1] that first described this new type of dwarfism, it was apparently not until 1968 that the term hitch-hiker's thumb was used to describe this peculiar clinical and radiographic finding[2].

Maurice Lamy and Pierre Maroteaux[1] wrote that first 1960 article and described three patients with what they named diastrophic (twisted) dwarfism. They emphasized that the findings of club feet, a thoracic (dorsal) scoliosis and a normal skull should allow one to differentiate this new condition from the most common form of dwarfism, achondroplasia, with which it might be confused. In 1968, Angel Vazquez and Fred Lee[2] (Children's Hospital of Pittsburgh) reported two additional cases. They used the term hitch-hiker's thumb in the radiographic description of the hand deformity of their second patient (Figure 1). 'The first metacarpal bones are markedly hypoplastic, and the thumbs appear low set and laterally directed in a 'hitch-hiker's' position.'[2]

The definition of hitch-hike is 'To travel by means of lifts in vehicles. Also 'hitch-hiker,' one who hitch-hikes.'[3] One gets a 'lift' by attracting the attention of a driver with the universal signal of the abducted and extended thumb (Figure 2).

References

1. Lamy, M. and Maroteaux, P. (1960). Le nanisme diastrophique. *Presse Med.*, 68, 1977–80

2. Vazquez, A.M. and Lee, F.A. (1968). Diastrophic dwarfism. *J. Pediatr.*, 72, 234–42

3. Hitch-hike. In Simpson, J. and Weiner, E. (eds.) *Oxford English Dictionary*, 1989, 2nd edn., Vol. 7, p. 266. (Oxford: Clarendon Press)

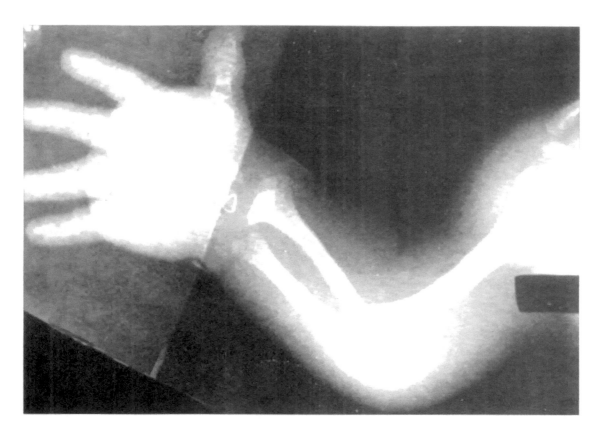

Figure 1. In patients with hitch-hiker's thumb 'the short tubular bones of the hands are variably dysplastic and the first metacarpal bones are characteristically shortened and rounded.' Reprinted from Vazquez and Lee[2]. Diastrophic dwarfism. *J. Pediatr.,* 1968, **72**, 234–42, with permission of Mosby-Year Book Inc.

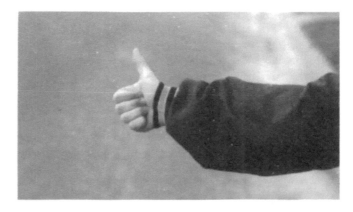

Figure 2. A hitch-hiker's thumb

HOCKEY STICK (FISHHOOK, J-SHAPED) URETER

The introduction of transurethral prostate resection and intravenous urography changed the clinical presentation and preoperative evaluation of patients with prostatic obstruction. Herman Kretschmer and Fay Squire[1] (Presbyterian Hospital, Chicago) recognized these changes and studied them in 408 patients seen from 1933–1947. Their primary goal was to study the frequency and extent of hydronephrosis in these patients with prostatic enlargement. In addition, they reported the radiographic changes seen in the course of the ureter. The 'changes consist[ed] of lateral displacement, angulation and elevation of the ureters at the point of their entrance into the bladder.'[1] In the figures illustrating the article, this is described as a 'fishhook course' (Figure 1). Many other terms including J-shaped or hockey stick (Figure 2) have also been used. (The hockey stick analogy was taught to me, during my medical student days, by Robert Spellman, a urologist at St Elizabeth's Hospital in Brighton, Massachusetts.) Kretschmer and Squire[1] emphasized that, 'The recognition of these changes in the ureters may be of diagnostic aid or value in some ... cases.' This sign is still valuable for recognizing prostate enlargement from either hypertrophy or tumor.

'It has been argued that the image of two figures holding sticks in a 'face off' position carved into early Egyptian pottery offers proof of a very early emergence of the game [of hockey].

The best available evidence suggests that ice hockey emerged out of various earlier games in Montreal [Canada] in the middle 1870s. Credit for the formulation of the original rules goes to J.G.H. Creighton, though evidence suggests that he did little more than organize an on-ice version of British field hockey.

The earliest reported hockey game was played on March 3rd, 1875. According to the Montreal Gazette, Creighton captained one of the sides.'[2]

References
1. Kretschmer, H.L. and Squire, F.H. (1948). The incidence and extent of hydronephrosis in prostatic obstruction. *J. Urol.*, 60, 1–6

2. Diamond, D. and Romain, J. (1988). *Hockey Hall of Fame*, p. 12. (New York: Doubleday)

Figure 1. 'Note high insertion of left ureter and fishhook course.' Reprinted from Kretschmer and Squire[1]. The incidence and extent of hydronephrosis in prostatic obstruction. *J. Urol.,* 1948, **60**, 1–6, with permission of Williams & Wilkins

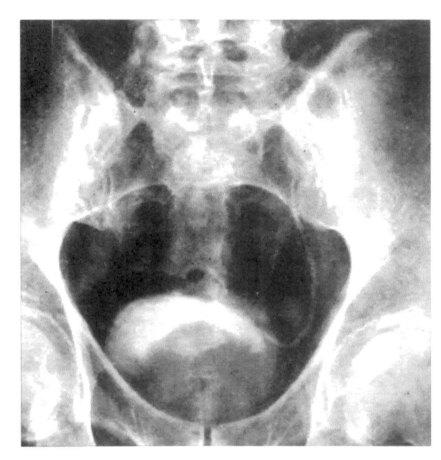

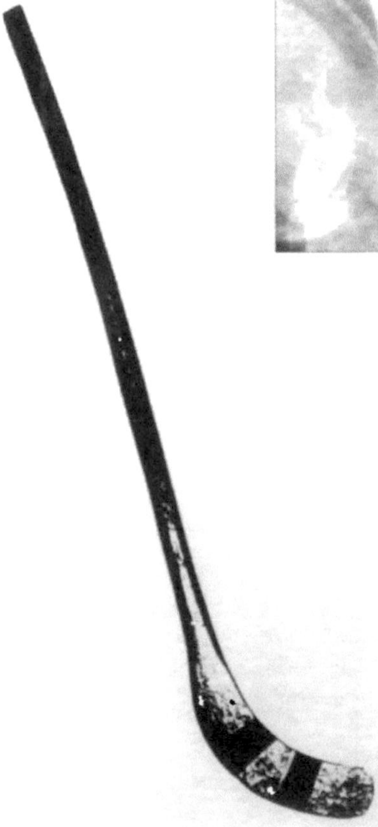

Figure 2. 'One of the sticks used in early hockey matches (circa 1860).'[2] Courtesy of Hockey Hall of Fame Archives

HONDA ('H') SIGN

Stress fractures and other stress phenomena are often detected with radionuclide bone scans before changes are evident on plain radiographs. The plain radiographic appearance may be very subtle or non-specific. In 1983, Todd Ries[1] (Baylor University Medical Center) reported a characteristic pattern, seen on radionuclide bone scans, in four patients with sacral insufficiency fractures. 'In each case, bone scans showed a characteristic H-shaped uptake pattern, with the central portion of radionuclide over the sacrum and the remainder over the sacroiliac joints.' The H-shaped pattern he described has become known as the Honda sign. The horizontal and vertical lines of increased uptake seen on the bone scan (Figure 1) indicate the areas of insufficiency fracture and resemble the letter H of the Honda automobile emblem (Figure 2). These insufficiency fractures can be a cause of pain in cancer patients. The fractures should not be confused with areas of metastatic disease. The Honda sign can now also be detected on computerized tomography and magnetic resonance imaging scans.

Soichiro Honda (1906–1991) established the Honda Technical Research Institute in October 1946. The company initially manufactured only small engines and motorbikes. In 1948 the firm was incorporated under the name Honda Motor Co. Ltd[2]. The American Honda Motor Company was formed in June 1959. That same year Honda motorcycles were sold in Los Angeles. In 1960 Honda began manufacturing cars in Japan. In 1969 they began selling their cars (the N600) in Hawaii, and then on the West Coast in 1970[3]. Specifics of the auto-emblem design remain shrouded in secrecy.

References
1. Ries, T. (1983). Detection of osteoporotic sacral fractures with radionuclides. *Radiology*, 146, 783–5

2. Sakiya, T. (1982). *Honda Motor – The Men, The Management, The Machines*, p. 7. (Tokyo: Kodansha International Ltd)

3. Shook, R.L. (1988). *Honda – An American Success Story*, pp. 30–6. (New York: Prentice Hall Press)

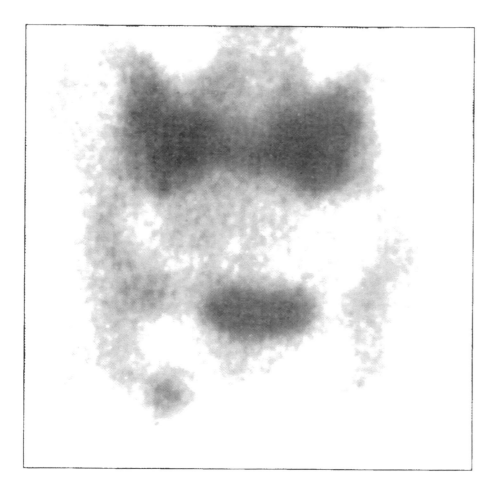

Figure 1. 'Posterior view of the pelvis shows the characteristic H-shaped pattern of uptake.' Reprinted from Ries[1]. Detection of osteoporotic sacral fractures with radionuclides. *Radiology*, 1983, **146**, 783–5 with permission of the RSNA

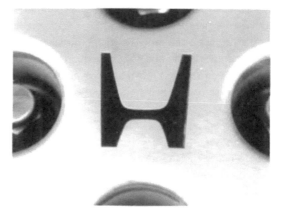

Figure 2. Honda automobile 'H'

HONEYCOMB LUNG

The book, *The Diseases of the Lungs*[1], was published in 1898. In the chapter, 'Bronchiectasis in Children,' Sir James Kingston Fowler and Rickman John Godlee used the term 'honeycomb appearance' in their description of the pathologic findings. Their discussion of the morbid anatomy was as follows: 'The lesions which specially characterize the most acute cases are: (a) acute peribronchitis; (b) dilatation of the bronchioles throughout extensive areas of the lungs, or almost the whole of both organs; (c) the presence of innumerable small cavities, which give the lungs a worm-eaten or honeycomb appearance; and (d) the presence on the surface of the lungs of small vesicles containing air.' Apparently the term worm-eaten did not catch on. They also stated, 'The exact pathology of the condition known as 'honeycomb lung' is not yet determined.' Today the term honeycomb lung is used by radiologists to describe any pathologic process leading to a chest radiographic appearance with multiple small (3–10 mm) thick-walled cystic spaces (Figure 1). The pattern also may be exquisitely shown using high resolution computerized tomographic scanning (Figure 2).

A honeycomb is the unique storage container of the honeybee (Figure 3). 'Appreciable [q]uantities of honey and wax can be obtained only from colonies of bees belonging to the single genus *Apis* and commonly known as honeybees ... Only four species of the genus are found in the world today.'[2] Only one is native to Europe and North America. Honeybees belong to the order Hymenoptera. 'The first true Hymenoptera to be discovered were found in rocks of the Jurassic period (150 million years old).'[2]

References
1. Fowler, J.K. and Godlee, R.J. (1898). *The Diseases of the Lungs*, pp. 143–9. (London: Longman's, Green and Co.)

2. Butler, C.G. (1962). *The World of the Honeybee*, pp. 3–11. (London: Collins Clear-Type Press)

3. Watts, B. (1989). *Honeybee*. (Englewood Cliffs, NJ: Silver Burdett Press)

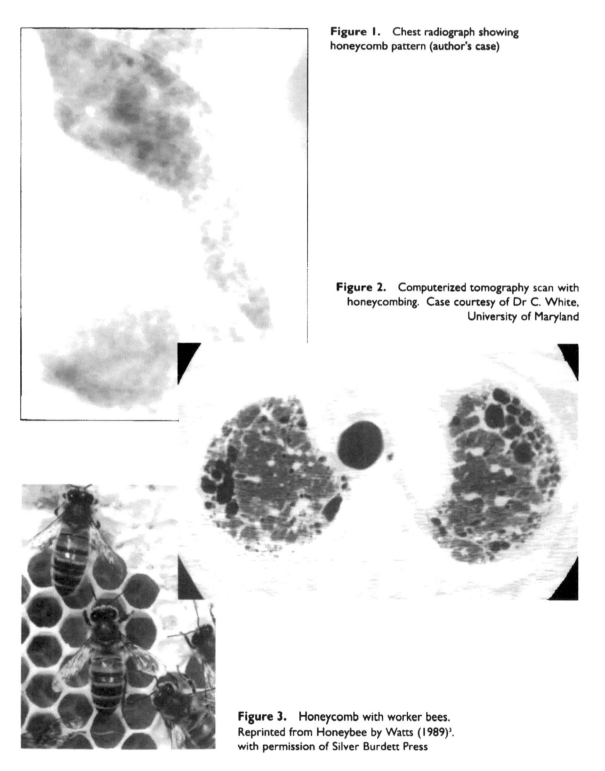

Figure 1. Chest radiograph showing honeycomb pattern (author's case)

Figure 2. Computerized tomography scan with honeycombing. Case courtesy of Dr C. White, University of Maryland

Figure 3. Honeycomb with worker bees. Reprinted from Honeybee by Watts (1989)³. with permission of Silver Burdett Press

HORSESHOE KIDNEY

Horseshoe kidney is the most common congenital fusion anomaly seen in the genitourinary system. It 'was described for the first time in 1522 by Berengario da Carpi [not by Vesalius (1514–1564) as others have stated] in the Isagogue, and the translation made by Jackson in 1660 reads:

> I myself also in the year of 1521 in our exercise at Bononia, saw in one publiquely Anatomised, ... in that individual the Kidneys were continued, as if it were one kidney; and it had two Veins, and two Emulgent arteries, and two Uritidian pores with only one Pannicle involving, which did take up the wonted places of the Kidneys, and also the middle part of the Back.

The condition was illustrated for the first time by Leonardo Botallo in 1564'[1] (Figure 1). Horseshoe kidney recognition is important because the kidney is more prone to trauma, urinary stasis, stone formation and obstruction with this condition (Figure 2).

'[I]t is still uncertain to whom ... we owe the invention of horse-shoeing (Figure 3). No Greek or Latin writer ... mentions shoeing with nailed on shoes. The Celts, however, are credited ... with having employed nailed-on shoes before the opening of the Christian era, and having extended their use throughout Gaul, Germany, and England. [I]n the East, the Mongols claim to have shod with iron since the earliest times.'[2]

References
1. Murphy, L.J.T. (1972). *The History of Urology*, p. 193. (Springfield, IL: Charles C. Thomas)

2. Dollar, J.N.O. (1898). *A Handbook of Horse-shoeing*, pp. 2–8. (Edinburgh: David Douglas)

Figure 1. The earliest illustration of horseshoe kidney. (From Botallo: *Commentarioli Duo*, Lugduni, 1565.) Reprinted from *The History of Urology* by Murphy (1972)[1]. Courtesy of Charles C. Thomas, Publisher, Springfield, IL

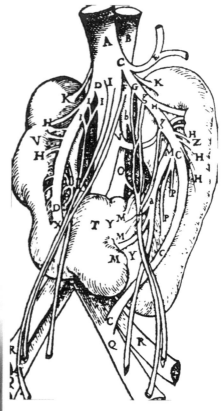

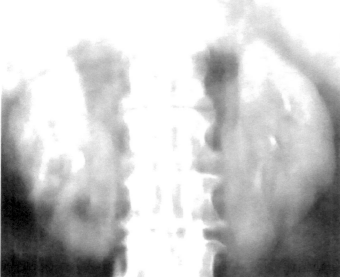

Figure 2. Nephrotomogram of horseshoe kidney. Case courtesy of Dr M. Severson, University of Maryland

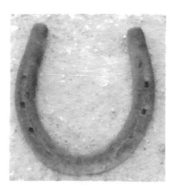

Figure 3. A horse's shoe

ICEBERG (TIP 0F THE ICEBERG) SIGN

Searching for pelvic masses with an ultrasound probe can be a difficult task; shadowing from bowel gas may obscure masses and some masses may obscure themselves. This fact is borne out in Paul Guttman's 1977 description[1] of benign cystic ovarian teratomas that showed only the 'tip of the iceberg'! He reported 23 surgically proven cases from Stanford University. '[T]he consistent, diagnostic feature was the presence of a complex mass with hyperechoic zones that produced acoustic shadowing of the far wall of the mass. In six cases ... only the near wall of the mass was recognized, hence the term 'tip of the iceberg' sign ... [T]he presence of highly reflective and attenuating hair within the sebaceous material ... produces [the] characteristic acoustic shadowing'[1] (Figure 1). He stressed the importance of not confusing this appearance with shadowing due to bowel gas and he discussed steps that could be taken to make the distinction. Today transvaginal ultrasound scanning, computerized tomography and magnetic resonance imaging make the diagnosis of pelvic masses a less hazardous task and pelvic 'icebergs' less of a danger.

'Ice in the waters of the Earth's polar regions occurs in two forms, namely, pack ice and icebergs. Pack ice forms from seawater and is generally only one to two years old, whereas icebergs are fragments of ice sheets and glaciers that formed on land areas during intervals of thousands of years [Figure 2]. ... Probably the first mention of icebergs was that of St Brendan [*circa* 489–583], an Irish monk whose partly fictional writings suggest that he encountered a 'floating crystal castle' on the high seas.'[2] These floating castles (icebergs) calve (break off) from glacier tips largely due to the ranging tides that intermittently increase and decrease the

'force on the protruding end of the glacier or ice shelf resulting in the birth of a large monolith of drifting ice.'[2,3]

References

1. Guttman, P.H. Jr (1977). In search of the elusive benign cystic ovarian teratoma: application of the ultrasound 'tip of the iceberg' sign. *J. Clin. Ultrasound*, 5, 403–6

2. Icebergs and pack ice. In *The New Encyclopaedia Britannica*, 1990, 15th edn, Vol. 20, p. 748. (Chicago: Encyclopaedia Britannica Inc)

3. O'Meara, J.J. (1976). *The Voyage of Saint Brendan: Journey to the Promised Land.* (Atlantic Highlands, NJ: Humanities Press Inc.)

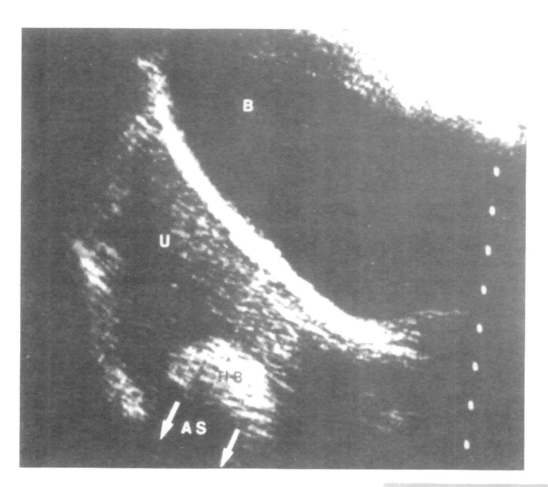

Figure 1. 'Midline sagittal sonogram demonstrating the near wall of the dermoid only due to acoustical shadowing (AS) from the hairball (HB), the so-called 'tip of the iceberg' sign.' Reprinted from Guttman[1]. In search of the elusive benign cystic ovarian teratoma. *J. Clin. Ultrasound*, 1977, **5**, 403–6. Copyright 1977 John Wiley & Sons. Reprinted by permission of John Wiley & Sons Inc.

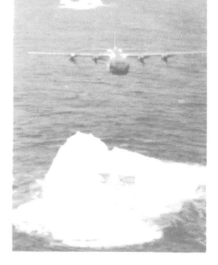

Figure 2. Icebergs in shipping lanes are monitored by patrol planes. Photograph courtesy of the US Coast Guard

IVORY VERTEBRA

The lead article in the *Revue Neurologique* in January 1925 was the report of the 'vertèbre d'ivoire' by Alexandre Souques and co-workers[1]. Their patient was a 57-year-old woman with breast cancer who had progressive weakening of her leg strength (or muscle strength). A radiographic examination of the thoracic spine showed a uniformly white T6 vertebra with no abnormality of its contour or adjacent disks (Figure 1). Lipiodol myelogram revealed a complete block at this level. They were reluctant to diagnose this abnormality as metastatic involvement since the patient had no other signs or symptoms of metastatic disease. (Oscar Batson's work demonstrating the venous connections to the paravertebral plexus from the deep pelvic veins and shoulder girdle would not be published until 1940[2].) Nevertheless their conclusion was that this ivory vertebra did indeed represent metastatic involvement. Joseph Récamier introduced the term metastasis to describe the spread of cancer in 1829[3]. Even today the two most common causes of ivory vertebrae are metastatic disease (especially from breast cancer and Hodgkin's disease) and Paget's disease.

Ivory, in elephant or walrus tusk, is a type of specialized tooth composed almost entirely of dentine. The upper canine teeth of the walrus and the upper incisors of the elephant elongate into their ivory tusks[4]. Figure 2 is a replica of a human lumbar vertebra carved from woolly mammoth tusk ivory.

References

1. Souques, A. A., Lafourcade, J. and Terris, E. (1925). Vertèbre 'd'ivoire' dans un cas de cancer metastatique de la colonne vertébrale. *Rev. Neurol.*, 32, 3–10

2. Batson, O.V. (1940). The function of the vertebral veins and their role in the spread of metastases. *Ann. Surg.*, 112, 138–49

3. Schmidt, J.E. (1959). *Medical Discoveries – Who and When*, p. 299. (Springfield, IL: Charles C. Thomas)

4. MacGregor, A. (1985). *Bone, Antler, Ivory and Horn*, p. 17. (London: Croom Helm Ltd)

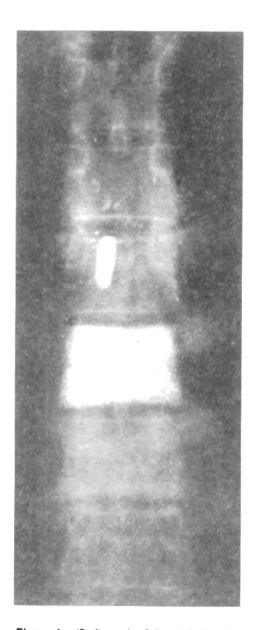

Figure 1. 'Radiograph of the sixth dorsal vertebra, white by convention and black on the film; this vertebra is remarkable for the integrity of its form and volume, and for the uniformity of its coloring.' (Film done 6 weeks after lipiodol myelogram.) Reprinted from Souques *et al.*[1] Vertèbre 'd'ivoire' dans un can de cancer metastatique de la colonne vertèbrale. *Rev. Neuvol.*, **32**, 3–10 with permission of Masson-Periodiques

Figure 2. Photograph (A) and radiograph (B) of carved ivory vertebra with comparison model vertebra. Ivory vertebra carved by D. O'Neill, T.C.R.'s Ivory, Fairbanks, Alaska. Specimen radiograph by J. Bode, Registered Radiologic Technologist (RRT)

A
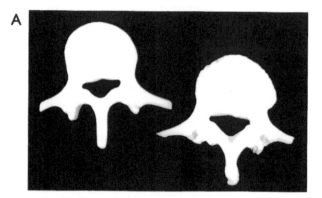

B
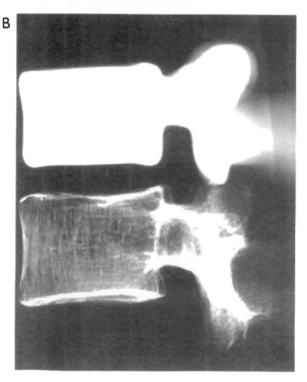

LEAD (GAS) PIPE SIGN

In 1923, the 'most common organic diseases of the colon [were] neoplasms, diverticulitis, tuberculosis, and chronic ulcerative colitis. The roentgenologic study of the colon in these conditions reveals obstruction of the bariumized medium, abnormal changes in its rate of passage, and transitory or constant deformities in the outline of the colon.'[1] The roentgenologic diagnosis of these common diseases was discussed in an article written by Russell Carman and Solomon Fineman[1] from the Mayo Clinic. Regarding the appearance of chronic ulcera-tive colitis they said, 'The characteristic roentgen-ray finding is a generalized narrowing of the lumen, which may be extreme in places. The contour of the bowel wall appears smooth and unhaustrated, resembling a gas pipe'[1] (Figure 1). The pipe analogy has persisted although the term 'lead pipe' seems to be used more commonly today. This sign is not pathognomonic for ulcerative colitis since other chronic inflammatory diseases of the colon also can result in a lead-pipe appearance on barium enema examinations.

Pipes used to transport gas to homes and businesses in the United States were originally made of lead (wrought iron was also used) (Figure 2). Thus, the two 'medical' terms are actually equivalent. 'In America, the distribution of manufactured gas through pipes began in 1816 as a public utility for lighting buildings and streets in Baltimore, MD [Maryland] ... The year 1825 marked the first commercial use of natural gas. At Fredonia, N.Y., gas was piped through small lead pipes.'[2]

References

1. Carman, R.D. and Fineman, S. (1923). The roentgenologic diagnosis of diseases of the colon. *Radiology*, 1, 129–42

2. Segeler, C.G. (1967). Gas-systems piping. In King, R.C. and Crocker, S. (eds) *Piping Handbook*, 5th edn, Chap. 13, p. 1. (New York: McGraw-Hill Book Co.)

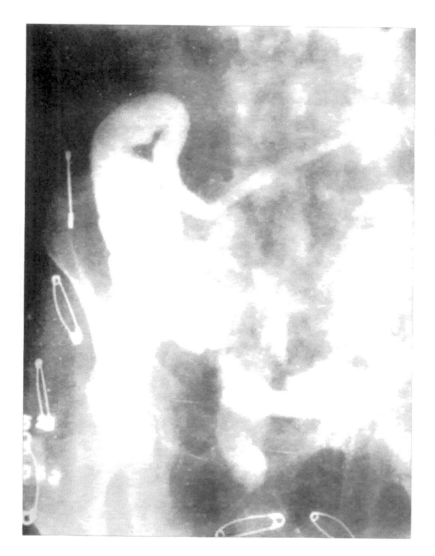

Figure 1. Lead-pipe sign seen in 'chronic ulcerative colitis. Note marked contraction of the colon.' Reprinted from Carman and Fineman[1]. The roentgenologic diagnosis of diseases of the colon. *Radiology*, 1923, 1, 129–42 with permission of the RSNA

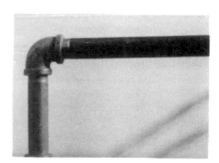

Figure 2. A gas pipe

LEMON AND BANANA SIGNS

Easily recognizable signs are useful to everyone. The lemon and banana signs were described in 1986 in the same article as 'two easily recognizable ultrasonographic signs that may be helpful both in screening for open spina bifida and in the evaluation of high-risk fetuses.'[1] These signs were observed during a retrospective review of 70 cases of open spina bifida performed in London, at the King's College Hospital, and were reported by Kypros Nicolaides and associates[1].

Detection of neural-tube defects is one aim of fetal ultrasound screening and maternal α-fetoprotein evaluation. However, the ultrasound examination of the fetal spine can be difficult and evaluation of the α-fetoprotein is not 100% sensitive or specific. The lemon sign refers to a scalloping of the frontal bones (Figure 1) that was seen in all cases of open spina bifida at the usual level for biparietal diameter measurement. The banana sign, an anterior curving of the cerebellar hemispheres (Figure 2), was seen in only 57% of cases. (Figure 3 shows a diagrammatic representation of the lemon and banana signs.) Neither of the signs was present in the control group of 100 patients.

Citrus is a genus of the family Rutaceae, with some 16 species that all have orange- or lemon-like fruits including the true lemon (*Citrus limon*, Figure 4). Records of citrus fruit cultivation can be found in China dating back to 2200 BC. Christopher Columbus is said to have introduced citrus fruit to the western hemisphere on his second voyage there in 1493[2].

Banana *(Musa sapientum)* belongs to the family Musaceae (Figure 5). It is a perennial tree-like herb. Its wild ancestors can still be found in the forests of Malaysia[2].

References

1. Nicolaides, K.H., Gabbe, S.G., Campbell, S. and Guidetti, R. (1986). Ultrasound screening for spina bifida: cranial and cerebellar signs. *Lancet*, ii, 72–4

2. Samson, J.A. (1986). *Tropical Fruits*, 2nd edn, pp. 73–8, pp. 139–43. (Essex: Longman Scientific and Technical)

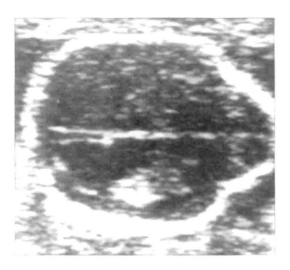

Figure 1. 'Transverse section of the fetal head at the level of the septum cavum pellucidum in an 18-week fetus with open spina bifida showing the lemon sign.' Reprinted from Nicolaides *et al.*[1] Ultrasound screening for spina bifida: cranial and cerebellar signs. *Lancet,* 1986, **ii,** 72–4, with permission of The Lancet Ltd

Figure 2. 'Suboccipital bregmatic view of the fetal head in an 18-week fetus with open spina bifida, showing the 'banana' sign (+).' Reprinted from Nicolaides *et al.*[1] Ultrasound screening for spina bifida: cranial and cerebellar signs. *Lancet,* 1986, **ii,** 72–74, with permission of The Lancet Ltd

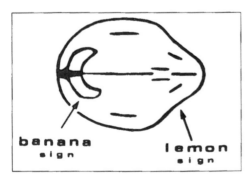

banana
sign

lemon
sign

Figure 3. Diagrammatic representation of the banana and lemon signs. Reprinted from Nicolaides *et al.*[1] Ultrasound screening for spina bifida: cranial and cerebellar signs. *Lancet,* 1986, **ii,** 72–4, with permission of The Lancet Ltd

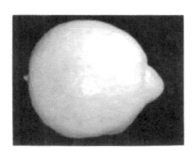

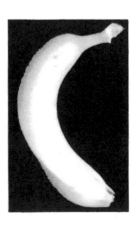

Figure 4. A lemon

Figure 5. A banana

LEONTIASIS OSSEA

Leontiasis is a descriptive term that has been used for at least three different disorders. The first use of the term was for a form of leprosy affecting the facial soft tissues. In this sense, the term has been used since Claudius Galen's time[1] (circa 130–201 AD). Second, the term was used for a type of elephantiasis affecting the soft tissues of the head and neck. Third, leontiasis ossea, was the name given by Rudolf Virchow (1821–1902) to a condition causing hyperostosis of the skull. He felt that the overgrowth of bone matched the elephantiasis of soft tissue and 'he decided to call these cases leontiasis ossea, not because the bone disease produced a leonine appearance, but because he considered it to be analogous to a disease of the soft parts which did.'[2] Virchow's description is based on the study of several skulls, the first one originally described by Marcello Malpighi (1628–1694) in the Opera Posthuma in 1700[2]. Another case known to Virchow, the first with a clinical history, is shown in Figure 2. Today, we use the term leontiasis ossea primarily to describe the skull changes due to the condition known as fibrous dysplasia (Figure 1). Whether any of the cases studied by Virchow were actually due to fibrous dysplasia is not known. Disorders other than fibrous dysplasia also give rise to leonine changes in facial bones. Among them are Paget's, renal osteodystrophy and reactive inflammatory bone disease[3].

'Animals that can be recognized as true cats are known from the early Pliocene. As far as the fossil record goes, big cats resembling lions and tigers turned up ... during the Villafranchian, as the early Pleistocene is called.'[4] During this ice age, the hunters of Europe depicted the lion *(Panthera leo)* on cave walls. 'It was then a cat of enormous size.'[4] Befitting the classic sign described above, a lion's head (and skull) is massive, thick and heavy (Figure 3).

References

1. Starr, M.A. (1894). Megalo-cephalie, or leontiasis ossea. *Am. J. Med. Sci.*, 18, 676–82

2. Knaggs, R.L. (1923). Leontiasis ossea. *Br. J. Surg.*, 11, 347–79

3. Lee, V.S., Webb, M.S., Martinez, S., McKay, C.P. and Leight, G.S. (1996). Uremic leontiasis ossea. *Radiology*, 199, 233–40

4. Guggisberg, C.A.W. (1975). *Wild Cats of the World*, pp. 19–20, pp. 139–40. (New York: Taplinger Publishing Co.)

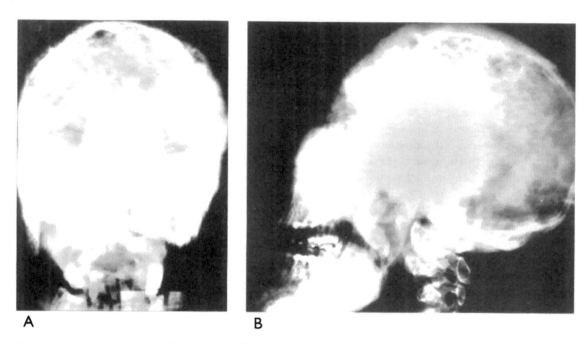

A   B

Figure 1. Anteroposterior (A) and lateral (B) views of the skull showing extreme deformation due to fibrous dysplasia. Case courtesy of Dr Anne Brower

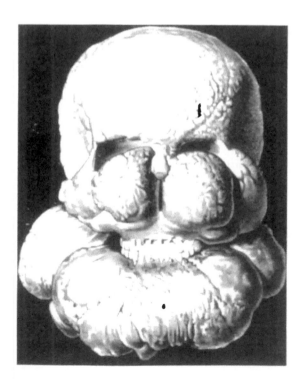

Figure 2. Drawing of Fourcade's case. The patient was his son who died at age 45 in 1767. Reprinted from Knaggs[2]. Leontiasis Ossea. *Br. J. Surg.*, 1923, 11, 347–79 with permission of Blackwell Science Ltd, the publisher

Figure 3. An African lion

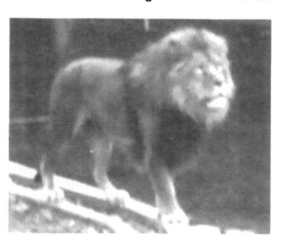

LINCOLN LOG (H-SHAPED) VERTEBRA

One hundred years after Abraham Lincoln's death, Jack Reynolds[1] reviewed the spinal changes in sickle cell disease at the sixty-sixth annual meeting of the American Roentgen Ray Society (September 28– October 1, 1965) held in Washington, DC. He considered usage of the term 'codfish vertebra' to describe the changes seen on spine radiographs of sickle cell patients unfortunate, since that term was originally intended to describe the spine changes of senile osteoporosis (see Codfish vertebra). 'The use of the term in this context [senile osteoporosis] was well established when, rather recently, it was first noted that cup-like depressions were present in the vertebral bodies of some patients with sickle cell disease'[1] (Figure 1). He said 'while the two types of deformities differ ... as yet, no substitute form of descriptive imagery has been fashioned to succinctly indicate the unique qualities of this stigma of the hemoglobinopathy.'[1] Later authors accepted this challenge and fashioned several descriptive terms such as step deformity[2], step-like[3], step-off and H-shaped[4]. During my radiology residency, I learnt to use the term Lincoln log to describe this vertebral body deformity that is due to infarction of the central portion of the growth plate. It is not pathognomonic for sickle cell disease, as it has been described in patients with thalassemia and in patients with Gaucher's disease. (Dr Reynolds agrees that the Lincoln log term is appropriate. He recalls that it was several years after his presentation when he first heard it used [Reynolds, personal communication].)

Lincoln Logs is a registered trademark of Playskool Inc. (Figure 2). This popular toy was 'designed and developed in 1916 by John Lloyd Wright, son of one of America's most famous architects, Frank Lloyd Wright. The younger Wright got his ideas for Lincoln Logs when he was with his father in Tokyo and saw the construction techniques used in the foundation of the earthquake-proof Imperial Hotel while it was being built'. He established the J.L. Wright Company and began manufacturing and selling this innovative construction toy.'[5]

Dr Henry Pritzker (Montefiore Hospital, New York) attributes the origin of this term to one of his mentors, Dr David Baker. Dr Baker recalls that he used the term when he taught at Babics Hospital, New York in the early 1960s likening the appearance of the short log connectors to the abnormal vertebral bodies (personal communications).

References

1. Reynolds, J. (1966). A re-evaluation of the 'fish vertebra' sign in sickle cell hemoglobinopathy. *Am. J. Roentgenol.*, 97, 693–707

2. Moseley, J.E. (1974). Skeletal changes in the anemias. *Semin. Roentgenol.*, 9, 169–84

3. Hansen, G.C. and Gold, R.H. (1977). Central depression of multiple vertebral end-plates: a pathognomonic sign of sickle hemoglobinopathy in Gaucher's disease. *Am. J. Roentgenol.*, 129, 343–4

4. Schwartz, A.M., Homer, M.J. and McCauley, R.G.K. (1979). 'Step-off' vertebral body: Gaucher's disease versus sickle cell hemoglobinopathy. *Am. J. Roentgenol.*, 132, 81–5

5. *Playskool History.* (Pawtucket, RI: Hasbro Inc.)

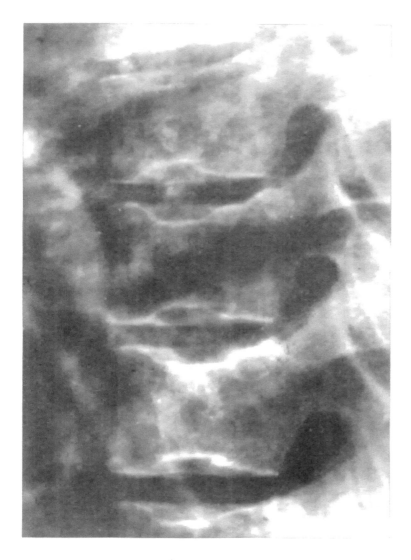

Figure 1. 'A portion of the thoracic spine of a young adult with sickle cell hemoglobinopathy in lateral projection. Near the center of each 'endplate,' the normal plane surface is deformed by a well defined, cup-like depression. Characteristically, both surfaces of each centrum exhibit identical depressions, and the shape of all of the involved segments is strikingly uniform.' Reprinted from Reynolds[1]. A re-evaluation of the 'fish vertebra' sign in sickle cell hemoglobinopathy. *Am. J. Roentgenol.*, **97**, 693–707, with the permission of the ARRS

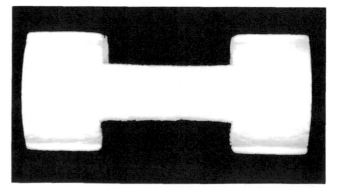

Figure 2. A Playskool Lincoln Log. Lincoln logs® is a registered trademark of Playskool Inc., Pawtucket, Rhode Island 02862. All rights reserved. Used with permission

LINGUINE (FREE-FLOATING LOOSE THREAD) SIGN

Imaging of the breast containing a silicone implant, used for augmentation mammoplasty or reconstruction after a mastectomy, was difficult before the invention of clinical magnetic resonance imaging (MRI). In the 1990s 'medical and public concern about the potential dangers of silicone leakage ... made it imperative to find a sensitive and specific diagnostic imaging modality for patients with silicone breast implants.'[1] David Gorczyca (University of California, Los Angeles) and his colleagues[1] evaluated various magnetic resonance pulse sequences in 143 patients to determine a reliable method for differentiating between silicone and normal breast tissue and to identify ruptures or leaks. One sign of an intracapsular rupture they described as the linguine sign or 'free-floating loose thread' sign. 'Pieces of free-floating silicone shell within the gel indicate an intracapsular rupture. We described this finding as the linguine sign or 'free-floating loose thread' sign.'[1] This indicates that there are free-floating pieces of the silicone shell within the silicone gel (Figure 1). This sign of intracapsular rupture should not be confused with normal radial folds that are present at the implant margin.

Pasta is any starchy food preparation made from semolina. It is formed into various special shapes (ribbons, cords, tubes) that were developed for specific characteristics, such as ability to hold a sauce or retain heat. Ribbon types include the narrow linguine (Figure 2) and the wider lasagna[3].

References

1. Gorczyca, D.P., Sinha, S., Ahn, C.Y. *et al.* (1992). Silicone breast implants *in vivo*: MR imaging. *Radiology*, 185, 407–10

2. Gorczyca, D.P., DeBruhl, N.D., Mund, D.F. and Bassett, L.W. (1994). Linguine sign at MR imaging: does it represent the collapsed silicone implant shell? *Radiology*, 191, 576–7

3. Pasta. In *The New Encyclopaedia Britannica*, 1990, 15th edn, Vol. 9, p. 188. (Chicago: Encyclopaedia Britannica Inc.)

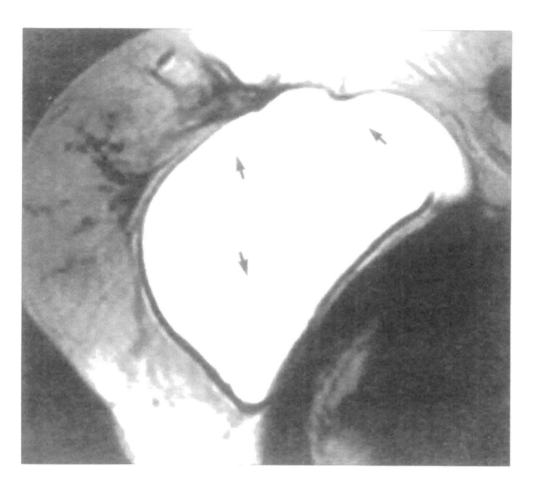

Figure 1. 'Intracapsular rupture. A 51-year-old woman presented with a 3-year history of severe chest and breast pain. Axial fast SE T2-weighted (4000/170, shoulder coil) image of the right breast obtained with water suppression demonstrates multiple curvilinear low-signal-intensity lines (arrows) within the high-signal-intensity silicone gel. These lines (linguine sign) represent the collapsed implant shell floating within the silicone gel.' Reprinted from Gorczyca et al.[1]. Silicone breast implants *in vivo*. *Radiology.*, 1992, **185**, 407–10, with permission of the RSNA

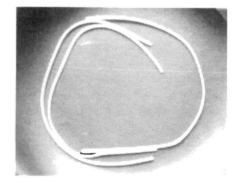

Figure 2. Linguine-19 pasta

MALLET (BASEBALL) FINGER

Mallet finger and baseball finger are the terms now used synonymously to depict the flexion deformity of the distal interphalangeal joint caused by rupture of the extensor tendon (Figure 1). Originally, however, they were used as opposites. Robert Abbe[1] (surgeon to St Luke's Hospital, New York) described 'two deformities of the end joint of the fingers ... which need the earliest surgical care' in 1894. The first (mallet finger) he called 'drop finger' finding that the 'extensor tendon ... had torn away from its delicate attachment to the base of the last joint.' The second (baseball finger) he said was the 'reverse deformity ... very commonly seen in baseball players. The last joint is violently dislocated backward and cannot be replaced, on account of the flexor tendons wrapping themselves round the head of the proximal bone of the joint.' British authors used the terms interchangeably as early as 1931. Harry Platt, senior surgeon at Ancoats Hospital, Manchester, said 'This injury has been frequently observed in baseball players and in cricketers ... the dropped phalanx and the lack of extension ... constitute the typical mallet finger.'[2] This injury can be seen in many different sports where the finger tip is subject to jamming or sudden bending including baseball, basketball, volleyball and football.

'The First Seeds that led to organized baseball in the United States were planted on the Elysian Fields in Hoboken, New Jersey, on June 19, 1846. Two amateur teams met and played a form of baseball no one had ever seen before. Under the rules established by Alexander J. Cartwright, a surveyor and amateur athlete, who umpired the game, the Knickerbockers were beaten by the New York Nine 23–1. Cartwright's game which included guidelines to the field as well as the playing rules, served to mark the only acceptable date of baseball's beginning. Before that, the origin is vague. Credit has been given to the Egyptians and every succeeding culture.'[3]

In Abbe's day, several different baseball associations competed with the National League for the fans' admission money of 25–50 cents. The true American League was formed in 1900 from the Western Association. The first 'World Series' was played in 1903 with the Boston Red Sox beating the Pittsburgh Pirates five games to three.

A mallet 'is a wooden variety of the malleus or hammer of the Romans ... it was in use in ancient times'[4] (Figure 2).

References
1. Abbe, R. (1894). The surgery of the hand. *N. Y. Med. J.*, 59, 33–40
2. Platt, H. (1931). Observations on some tendon ruptures. *Br. Med. J.*, i, 611–15
3. The Development of Baseball. *The Baseball Encyclopedia*, 1976, 3rd edn, pp. 9–13. (New York: Macmillan Publishing Co. Inc.)
4. Mercer, H.C. (1960). *Ancient Carpenter's Tools*, p. 171. (Doylestown, PA: Bucks County Historical Society)

Figure 1. Typical radiographic appearance of mallet finger (author's case)

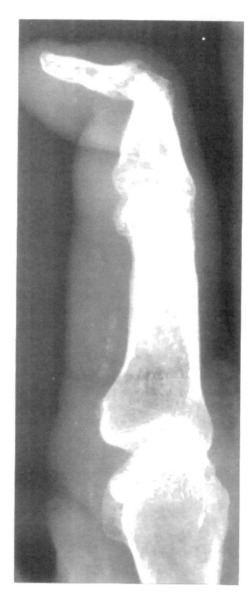

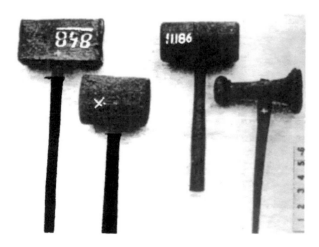

Figure 2. 'The carpenter's mallet.' Reprinted from *Ancient Carpenter's Tools* by Mercer (1960)[4], with permission of the Bucks County Historical Society, Doylestown, Pennsylvania

MARBLE BONE

Marble bone disease was first described by Heinrich Albers-Schönberg[1] (1865–1921) in 1904. Fritz Schulze[2] coined the term marmorknochen (marble bone) in 1921. Albers-Schönberg's patient was a 23-year-old merchant whose diffuse osteosclerosis (Figure 1) was said to give the bones a 'marble-like' appearance. He was first seen after a stumble in a hole caused a femur fracture. Roentgenograms revealed an 'ebony' appearance of the femur (due to the 'reverse', black bone on white background, printing) with no evidence of a medullary space. Further examination of the whole skeleton revealed the diffuse osteosclerosis that Albers-Schönberg[3] described, as if 'formed from marble', in his second report on the same patient. Our current term for this hereditary disorder of osteoblasts is osteopetrosis or Albers-Schönberg disease. At the time of the first report an increase in bone density was often attributed to an increase in the 'lime content of the bones.' Perhaps this is one of the reasons the term marble bone was chosen since 'marble is a limestone which has crystallized through heat and pressure.'[4] There are very few other disorders in young patients that can cause such a diffuse homogeneous increase in bone density. One key to the diagnosis of osteopetrosis is an inability to distinguish the normal boundary between the medullary space and the cortex. This important point was mentioned by Albers-Schönberg in his original report.

'Marble pieces date to the third millennium BC ... [b]ut it was not until the 7th and 6th century BC that the Greeks began to use white marble systematically, both for sculpture and for architecture.'[4] Figure 2 shows an example of a white-marble sculpture.

References

1. Albers-Schönberg, H. (1904). Röntgenbilder einer seltenen Knochenerkrankung. *Aerztlicher Verein*, Feb.

2. Schulze, F (1921). Das Wesen des Krankenheitsbildes der 'Marmorknochen (Albers-Schönberg)'. *Arch. Klin. Chir.*, 118, 411–38

3. Albers-Schönberg, H. (1907). Eine bisher nicht beschriebene Allgemeinerkrankung des Skeletts im Röntgenbild. *Fortschr. Geb. Röntgenstr.*, 11, 261–3

4. Ward-Perkins, J.B. (1992). In Dodge, H. and Ward-Perkins, B. (eds) *Marble in Antiquity, Collected Papers of J.B. Ward-Perkins*, pp. 13–20. (London: The British School at Rome)

5. Enggass, R. (1976). *Early Eighteenth-Century Sculpture In Rome*. (University Park, PA: Pennsylvania State University Press)

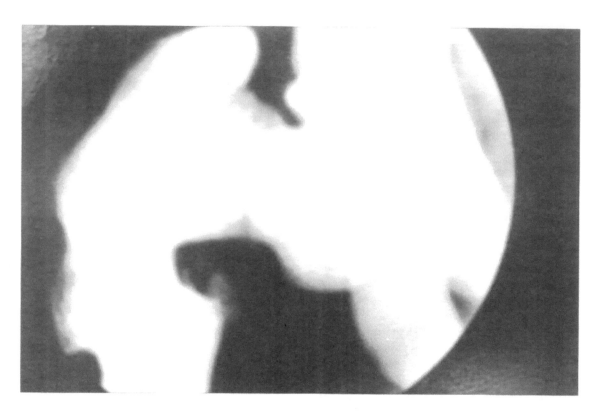

Figure 1. Anteroposterior radiograph of Albers-Schönberg's patient showing healed femoral fracture and uniformly dense (marble) bone. Reprinted from Albers-Schonberg[1]. *Röntgenbilder einer seltenen Knochenerkrankung. Aerztlicher Verein,* 1904, **Feb**

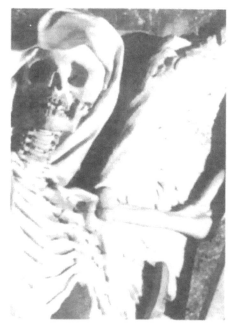

Figure 2. White marble sculpture (detail from Le Gros, Monument to Cardinal Cinzio Aldobrandini, *1707, S. Pietro in Vincoli).* Reproduced from Figure 134. *Early Eighteenth-Century Sculpture In Rome* by Enggass (1976)[5], published by Pennsylvania State University Press. Copyright 1976 by The Pennsylvania State University. Reproduced by permission of the publisher

MERCEDES–BENZ (MERCEDES STAR) SIGN

Before the advent of cholecystography and ultrasound, the diagnosis of gallstones was difficult to make. Seventy-five to 85% of gallstones are not radiopaque. Fissures within gallstones have been known to pathologists for more than 200 years[1]. The first depiction of these fissures is said to have been made by Walter[2] in 1796. They were first written about, in the medical literature, in 1931 by Karl Bauer[3] and Breuer[4]. The latter used the term 'star sign' to describe the pattern of fissuring evident on plain radiographs. H.R.C. Hay[5] attributed the phrase 'Mercedes-Benz' sign to the 1938 paper written by Burkhard Kommerell and Carlheinrich Wolpers[6] (Universitätsklinik der Charité, Berlin). The actual term used by Kommerell and Wolpers was 'Mercedes star' (Mercedesstern). Recognition of this triradiate gas pattern (Figure 1) allows the diagnosis of cholelithiasis to be made even when the stone is only faintly visible. One must be careful not to mistake gas trapped within the folds of the gastric pylorus for the fissures in a gallstone.

The car companies begun by Carl Benz (1844–1929) and Gottlieb Daimler (1834–1900) merged in June 1926 to become Daimler–Benz Aktiengesellschaft or Daimler–Benz AG. Each of the original two companies had a distinct emblem for their automobiles. The new company emblem combined the Mercedes (Daimler) three-point star with the Benz laurel wreaths as shown in Figure 2.

Austrian businessman Emil Jellinek, one of Daimler's board of directors, named the new line of Daimler cars introduced in 1900, 'Mercedes', after his 10-year-old daughter. The Mercedes three-point star was developed in 1909, modified in 1916 and, as it appears on today's cars (Figure 3), was patented in 1921[7]. The three points of the Mercedes star symbolize Daimler's involvement in the production of three modes of transportation – cars, ships and airplanes. The Benz laurel wreaths are said to signify the victory wreaths bestowed on their winning race car drivers.

References

1. Schwarz, G.S. (1952). Gas-containing gallstones. *Med. Radiogr. Photogra.*, 28, 72–4

2. Walter, F.A. (1796). *Anatomisches Museum.* (Berlin)

3. Bauer, K.H. (1931). Über selbstzertrümmerung von Gallensteinen und Neubildung von Steinen auf der Grundlage von Steintrümmern. *Arch. Klin. Chir.*, 165, 53–80

4. Breuer, B. (1931). Ueber das neues Röntgensymptom der Gallensteinkrankheit. *Röntgenpraxis*, 3, 879–81

5. Hay, H.R.C. (1966). Gas in gall stones: a rare radiological sign in the acute abdomen. *Gut*, 7, 387

6. Kommerell, B. and Wolpers, C. (1938). Gashaltige Gallensteine. *Fortschr. Geb. Röntgenstr.*, 58, 156–74

7. Robson, G. (1984). In *Mercedes-Benz. The First Hundred Years*, pp. 4–20. (Skokie, IL: Consumer Guide)

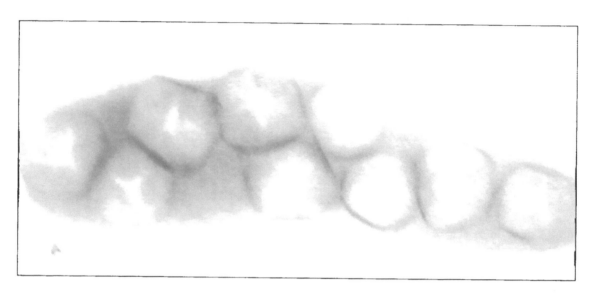

Figure 1. Resected specimen showing the Mercedes–star sign. 'The gas filled cracks are especially well seen.' Reprinted from Kommerell and Wolpers[5]. Gashaltige Gallensteine. *Fortschr. Geb. Rontgenstr.,* 1938, **58,** 156–174, with permission of Georg Thieme Verlag

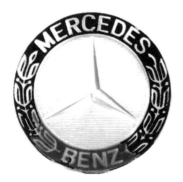

Figure 2. Mercedes–Benz emblem

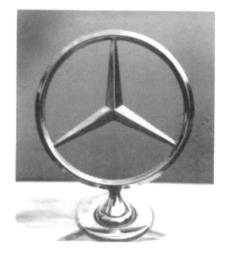

Figure 3. Mercedes hood ornament

MICKEY MOUSE SIGN

Real-time free-hand ultrasound scanning is one of the current indispensable imaging tools. Training radiology residents and technologists (ultrasonographers) how to do ultrasound examinations can be a challenge. Royal Bartrum and Harte Crow are two of the best teachers of this craft. Their book, *Real-Time Ultrasound*, is an excellent introductory text. One of the practical points they illustrated in the book is the Mickey Mouse sign (Figure 1). They used this sign to help residents and others find the common bile duct more easily. Prior to their description, longitudinal scanning with attempts to trace the hepatic vascular and biliary ductal structures was the norm, but this was often confusing. The Mickey Mouse sign, seen in transverse scans, was more easily reproducible (Bartrum, personal communication). 'The portal vein is Mickey Mouse's face, the main bile duct is his right ear, and the hepatic artery his left ear. Once you have this relationship in mind, it is no trick to find the duct [main bile duct] quickly in nearly every patient.'[1]

Mickey was introduced in 1928 in 'Steamboat Willie'. This was the first animated cartoon with sound. Mickey was created by Walt Disney and customarily drawn by Ub Iwerks, although his voice was provided by Disney himself until 1946[2]. (Unfortunately, the Walt Disney Co. would not grant permission for an official image of the famous mouse to be reproduced here.)

References
1. Bartrum, R.J. and Crow, H.C. (1983). *Real-Time Ultrasound*, p. 100. (Philadelphia: W.B. Saunders Co.)

2. Mickey Mouse. In *The New Encyclopaedia Britannica*, 1990, 15th edn, Vol. 8, p. 100. (Chicago: Encyclopaedia Britannica Inc.)

3. Bartrum, R. J. and Crow, H. C. (1980). Inflammatory diseases of the biliary system. Semin. in USD, 1, 102–8

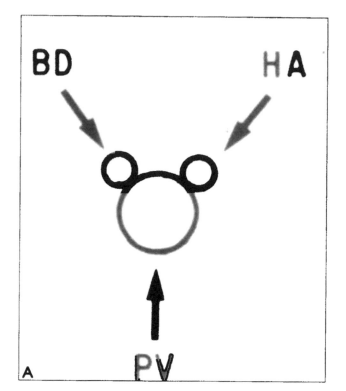
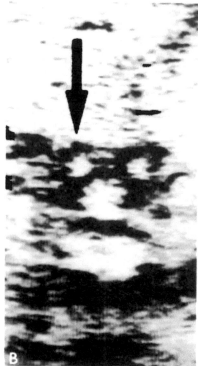

Figure 1. (A) A cross-section of the porta hepatis resembles Mickey Mouse (PV, portal vein; HA, hepatic artery; BD, main bile duct). (B) The transverse or 'Mickey Mouse' view is the easiest way to identify the main bile duct (arrow). Reprinted from Bartrum and Crow[3]. Inflammatory diseases of the biliary system. *Semin. in USD*, 1980, 1, 102–8, with the permission of the author and W.B. Saunders Company

MILIARY PATTERN

A miliary pattern, as seen on a chest radiograph, refers to the presence of multiple tiny (1–3 mm) nodular opacities scattered diffusely throughout the lung parenchyma (Figure 1). In *Stedman's Medical Dictionary*[1], the word miliary is defined as 'resembling a millet seed in size.' The term has its origins in the *Sepulchretum*[2], a book republished by Jean Jacques Manget (1652–1742) in 1700. The *Sepulchretum* is a collection of autopsy cases with pathologic descriptions. Manget, a Prussian physician, added several of his own cases to those already published by Theophilus Bonetus (1620–1689) of Geneva. One of Manget's cases was a 17-year-old lad who had died of tuberculosis (TB). The tubercles throughout the lungs, liver, spleen and mesentery were described by Manget as the size of millet seeds (magnitudine seminum milii)[3]. The seed analogy may relate to Heironymous Frascatorius' 1546 theory, published in his *De Contagione,* that 'imperceptible particles or 'seminaria', the seeds of disease ... could exist outside the body for several years and still infect.'[4]

Francis Henry Williams (1852–1936) of Boston City Hospital, 'America's first radiologist' was certainly one of the first to see a miliary pattern using roentgen rays. He discussed the use of the fluoroscope in diagnosis of diseases of the thorax (including TB) in the April 30, 1896 issue of the *Boston Medical and Surgical Journal* (precursor to the *New England Journal of Medicine*)[5]. He also wrote about the value of fluoroscopy and the X-ray examination in cases of pulmonary TB, including the miliary form, in an 1899 article and in his 1901 textbook, *The Roentgen Rays in Medicine and Surgery*[6,7].

'Millet is, any of various grasses, members of the Gramineae (Poaceae) family, producing small [1–3 mm] edible seeds [Figure 2] used as forage crops and as food cereals. Millets [were] probably first cultivated in Asia or Africa more than 4000 years ago ... they were major grains in Europe during the Middle Ages. About 30 million metric tons of millet are produced annually.'[8]

References
1. Milary. *Stedman's Medical Dictionary,* 1976, 23rd edn, p. 876. (Baltimore: Williams and Wilkins)

2. Manget, J.J. (1700). *Sepulchretum;sive, Anatomia practica, ex cadaveribus morbo denatis, proponens historias et observationes omnium humani corporis affectuum.* (Geneva: Sumptibus Cramer & Perachon)

3. Webb, G.B. (1936). *Tuberculosis,* pp. 63–4. (New York: P.B. Hoeber Inc.)

4. Rubin, S. A. (1995). Tuberculosis. *Radiol. Clin. North Am.,* 33, 619–39

5. Brecher, R. and Brecher, E. (1969). Francis, H., Williams: America's first radiologist. In *The Rays: A History of Radiology in the United States and Canada,* pp. 70–2. (Baltimore: Williams and Wilkins)

6. Williams, F.H. (1899). Röntgen-ray examinations in incipient pulmonary tuberculosis. *Trans. Am. Climat. Assoc.,* 15, 68–86

7. Williams, F.H. (1901). *The Roentgen Rays in Medicine and Surgery,* pp. 125–57. (London: Macmillan Co.)

8. Millet. In *The New Encyclopaedia Britannica,* 1990, 15th edn, Vol. 8, p. 137. (Chicago: Encyclopaedia Britannica Inc.)

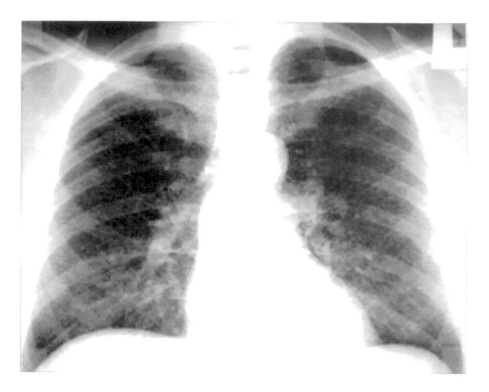

Figure 1. Chest radiograph of patient with miliary tuberculosis. Case courtesy of Dr M. Lesar, Bethesda Naval Hospital

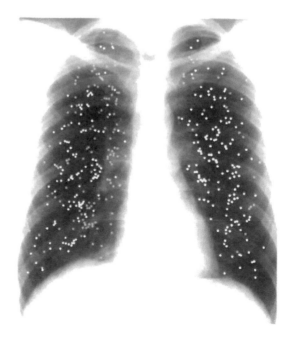

Figure 2. Chest radiograph with millet seeds superimposed

MOGUL SHADOW

'Skiagraphing the Mediasternal Moguls'[1] was a somewhat tongue in cheek 1970 review of roentgen cardiac diagnosis by Marvin Daves, then Professor and Chairman of the Department of Radiology, University of Colorado Medical Center. Daves, now retired, used to be an avid skier who frequented the Winter Park area in Colorado (personal communication). The article's title is a word play that cleverly links one of the early terms for a radiograph (skiagraph [shadow-picture]) to his subject. The word mediastinal was inadvertently misspelled in the title of the article (Daves, personal communication).

The moguls (Figure 1) are the prominent rounded shadows cast by the various mediastinal vascular and cardiac structures (first mogul, aorta; second mogul, pulmonary artery; third mogul, left atrial appendage; fourth mogul, cardiac apex). Daves reminded us that specific criteria must be met to equate these 'little hills' with their vascular counterparts. The article emphasized the appearance of the third mogul. Thus, it is this term that has persisted as one of our classics. When the third mogul is seen (together with enlargement of the second, as Daves taught), it is a reliable sign of enlargement of the left atrial appendage and is most often a manifestation of rheumatic heart disease.

Simply stated, moguls are snow bumps. They can occur naturally or can be man-made purposefully to make a ski slope more challenging (Figure 2). Mogul skiing became an Olympic event, as part of the demonstration sport called freestyle skiing, at the Calgary games in 1988. Freestyle skiing became a full medal sport at the 1992 games held in Albertville, France[2].

References
1. Daves, M. (1970). Skiagraphing the mediasternal moguls. *New Physician*, 19, 48–54
2. Connors, M., Dupuis, D., MacNee, M.J. and Brelin, C. (1994). *The Olympic Factbook – A Spectator's Guide to the Winter Games*, p. 201. (Detroit: Visible Ink Press)

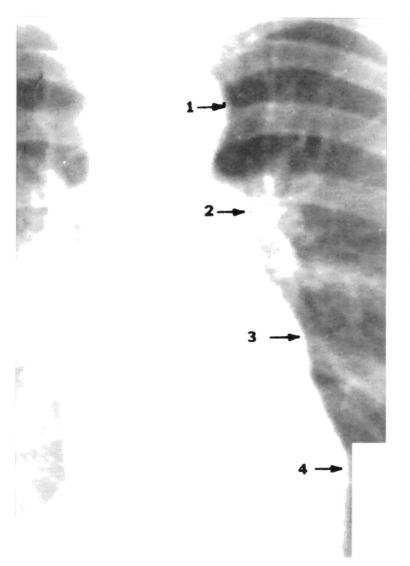

Figure 1. 'Mitral stenosis illustrating the four left moguls. First mogul [aorta] is above the carina, second mogul [main pulmonary artery] just above the left main stem bronchus, third mogul [left atrial appendage] just below the left main stem bronchus, and fourth mogul [cardiac apex] sits on the dome of the left hemidiaphragm.' Reprinted from Daves'. Skiagraphing the mediasternal moguls. *New Physician*, 1970, **19**, 48–54, with permission from *The New Physician*, copyright 1970, American Medical Student Association

Figure 2. Skier on mogul slope

MOTH-EATEN PATTERN

One early definition of the moth eaten pattern of bone destruction was given by Webster Belden[1] (New York Hospital) in 1925. While describing a case of multiple myeloma, he said, 'The lesions are multiple and the bones are pierced by small focal spots of destruction which are not confluent.'[1] Although Belden did not use the term moth eaten, Ernest Codman[2] used it that same year, to describe the radiographic appearance of multiple myeloma, which 'may at times show invasion of the bone in a moth-eaten way.' This pattern of destruction is not specific for myeloma since it can be seen with many other aggressive primary bone tumors and at times with aggressive non-neoplastic conditions like osteomyelitis (Figure 1).

Various patterns of bone destruction give valuable clues regarding the biological activity of the underlying process. We are indebted to the organizers of the Bone Tumor Registry (Codman, James Ewing, Joseph Bloodgood) for the early foundation of this knowledge (see Codman triangle for the history of the Registry). Among others, special recognition must be given to Gwilym Lodwick and Lent Johnson. While working at the Armed Forces Institute of Pathology (AFIP) in Washington, DC, they codified and defined, once and for all, the terms used to describe bone tumors. Their work allows us to use the terms geographic, moth-eaten and permeative destruction with precision. They carefully analyzed and correlated the radiographic, gross pathologic and macrosection findings of the bone tumor cases in the AFIP files. This original work was presented at the Radiological Society of North America meeting in 1951[3] and at the American Roentgen Ray Society meeting in 1954[4]. Although it was accepted for publication in the American Journal of Roentgenology, final permission to publish it was not given and the original work remains in the realm of unpublished data (Lodwick, personal communication). Thankfully, much of this material has been published in subsequent books and papers[5-8](Figure 2).

Moths and butterflies form the order Lepidoptera (Figure 3). 'The name is derived from the Greek words [for] 'scale,' and, 'wing,' referring to the scales covering the surfaces of the wings; the structure and pigments of these scales are responsible for the extraordinary variety of wing colours.'[9] There are about 165 000 species in the order Lepidoptera. 'Fossil species ... have been found in amber ... dat[ing] from the lower Cretaceous, some 100 to 130 million years [ago].'[9]

References
1. Belden, W.W. (1925). A case report of multiple myeloma. Am. J. Roentgenol., 13, 442–7
2. Codman, E.A. (1925). The nomenclature used by the registry of bone sarcoma. Am. J. Roentgenol., 13, 105–26
3. Lodwick, G.S. and Johnson, L.C. (1951). Primary sarcomas of bone, integration of radiologic and pathologic observations. Presented at the Radiological Society of North America, Chicago, IL, December
4. Lodwick, G.S. and Johnson, L.C. (1954). Roentgen evaluation of malignant bone tumors. Presented at the American Roentgen Ray Society, Washington, DC, September
5. Lodwick, G.S. (1971). The Bones and Joints, pp. 6–64. (Chicago: Year Book Medical Publishers)
6. Madewell, J.E., Ragsdale, B.D. and Sweet, D.E. (1981). Radiologic and pathologic analysis of solitary bone lesions. I: Internal margins. Radiol. Clin. North Am., 19, 715–48
7. Ragsdale, B.D., Madewell, J.E. and Sweet, D.E. (1981). Radiologic and pathologic analysis of solitary bone lesions. II: Periosteal reactions. Radiol. Clin. North Am., 19, 749–83
8. Sweet, D.E., Madewell, J.E. and Ragsdale, B.D. (1981). Radiologic and pathologic analysis of solitary bone lesions. III: Matrix patterns. Radiol. Clin. North Am., 19, 785–814
9. Sbordoni, V. and Forestiero, S. (1984). Butterflies of the World, p.12. (New York: Times Books)

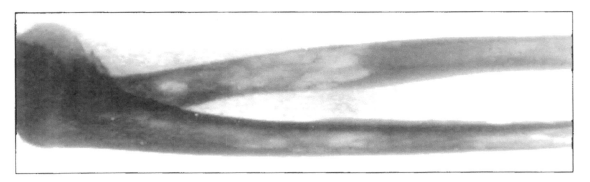

Figure 1. Moth eaten pattern of destruction. From *The Bones and Joints* by Lodwick (1971)[5], published by Year Book Medical Publishers, Chicago. Copyright 1971 with ACR. Reprinted with permission

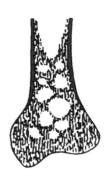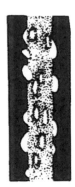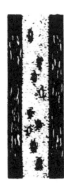

Figure 2. Moth eaten (A and B) and permeative (C) patterns of destruction. Reprinted from Madewell *et al.*[4] Radiologic and pathologic analysis of solitary bone lesions. 1: Internal margins. *Radiol. Clin. North Am.*, 1981, **19**, 715–48, with permission of WB Saunders Company

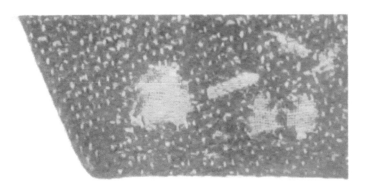

Figure 3. 'Work of clothes moths'. Reprinted from *Injurious Insects* by O'Kane, W.C. (1912), published by The Macmillan Company, New York

NAPOLEON HAT (BOW) SIGN

Sir James Brailsford[1] (The Queen's Hospital, London) discussed many deformities of the lumbosacral spine in a lengthy 1929 article. One of the conditions he elaborated on was spondylolisthesis. Regarding the antero-posterior radiographs he said, 'These may be absolutely typical ... It will be seen that the anterior border of the transverse process is continuous with the anterior border of the body. With a definite case of spondylolisthesis, the superior surface of the body of the 5th lumbar vertebra is facing forwards, and an antero-posterior radiograph of the patient will show the 5th lumbar body and transverse processes in this plane, and this characteristic outline [Figure 1] of the anterior border of the body and transverse processes will be projected against the shadow of the sacrum.' He later used the term 'bow sign' to describe this appearance[2]. Other terms, more commonly used today, include the Napoleon hat sign or gendarme's hat sign (the latter from Anne Brower, personal communication).

'The term spondylolisthesis or gliding vertebra was first used by Killian in 1853. The condition itself had previously been mentioned by Herbineau in 1782, Rokitanski in 1839 and Belloc in 1849.'[3]

Napoleon Bonaparte (1769–1821) was one of the greatest military men in French history. He became a general at age 24, a commander-in-chief at age 27, and Emperor of France at age 35. Leading troops on the battlefield, he was not usually given to extravagant dress[4]. The bicorne hat supplanted the tricorne in the 1790s and became Napoleon's 'signature hat'[5] (Figure 2).

References
1. Brailsford, J.F (1929). Deformities of the lumbosacral region of the spine. Br. J. Surg., 16, 562–627

2. Brailsford, J.F. (1934). The Radiology of Bones and Joints, p. 286. (London: J & A Churchill)

3. Garland, L.H. and Thomas, S.F. (1946). Spondylolisthesis. Am. J. Roentgenol., 55, 275–91

4. Bonaparte, N. (1992). In De Chair, S. (ed.) Napoleon on Napoleon: An Autobiography of the Emperor, pp. 12–19. (London: Cassell)

5. McDowell, C. (1992). Hats: Status, Style and Glamour, pp. 13–32. (London: Thames and Hudson)

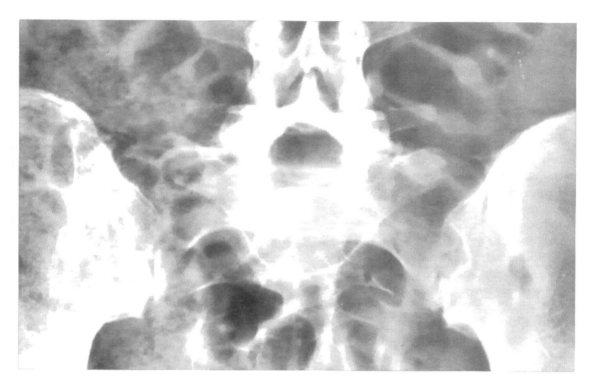

Figure 1. Anteroposterior radiograph showing Napoleon-hat sign of spondylolisthesis. Case courtesy of Dr C. Resnik, University of Maryland

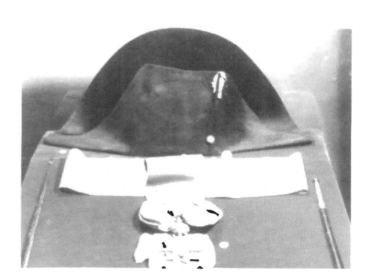

Figure 2. One of Napoleon's hats on exhibit at Musée de l'Armée, Paris. (Worn by Napoleon at the battle of Eylau, February 8, 1807)

ONION SKIN SIGN

James Ewing's original description[1] (1921) of the diffuse endothelioma of bone, that is now called Ewing's tumor, did not include the pungent term (onion skin) later used to depict the layers of periosteal reaction often seen when this tumor penetrates the cortex of a long bone (Figure 1). Ernest Amory Codman[2] did use the term in his 1925 article that presented the 'official nomenclature' of the Registry of Bone Sarcoma, when he said, 'Roentgenologically it shows a characteristic longitudinal striation and the tumor nearly always involves more than half of the shaft. It does not often produce the radiating spicules, [see Sunburst sign] but there may be onion-like layers of periosteal new-bone formation such as one sees in osteomyelitis.'[2] We do not know which of the contributors* to the 'official nomenclature' first used the term in reference to Ewing's tumor. Ewing (1866–1943) never uses it in any of the editions of his book, *Neoplastic Diseases; A Treatise on Tumors*[3]. The latest edition appeared in 1940. Regarding the name 'Ewing's tumor' Codman said, 'As a matter of classification we carry this tumor under Ewing's name, rather against his will and more or less to his mortification, because he not infrequently disowns a tumor which the Registrar [Codman] tries to place under his name.'[2]

Layered or laminated periosteal reaction (onion-skin) was reported, in the Intergroup Ewing's Sarcoma Study, to be a common finding in cases of Ewing's tumor. It was present in 198 of the 350 cases (56.6%)[4]. Codman also pointed out that a layered periosteal reaction can be seen in cases of osteomyelitis. Other entities that may show a layered periosteal reaction include osteosarcoma and Langerhans cell histiocytosis (eosinophilic granuloma). The term onion skin is not usually applied until three distinct layers of periosteal reaction are evident.

Onion *(Allium cepa)*, is a 'herbaceous biennial plant [or] its edible bulb [Figure 2]. Probably native to southwestern Asia, the plant belongs to the lily family, Liliaceae. Onions are among the world's oldest cultivated plants.'[5]

---

*E.A. Codman (Boston), J. Ewing (New York), J.C. Bloodgood (Baltimore), W.C. MacCarty (Mayo Clinic), F.E. Sondern (New York), A.V. St George (New York) and H.H. Bell (Minneapolis).

References

1. Ewing, J. (1921). Diffuse endothelioma of bone. *Proc. New York Pathol. Soc.*, 21, 17–24

2. Codman, E.A. (1925). The nomenclature used by the Registry of Bone Sarcoma. *Am. J. Roentgenol.*, 13, 105–26

3. Ewing, J. (1940). *Neoplastic Diseases; A Treatise on Tumors*, 4th edn. (Philadelphia: Saunders)

4. Reinus, W.R. and Gilula, L.A. (1984). Radiology of Ewing's sarcoma: Intergroup Ewing's Sarcoma Study (IESS). *Radio Graphics*, 4, 929–44

5. Onion. In *The New Encyclopaedia Britannica*, 1990, 15th edn, Vol. 8, p. 955. (Chicago: Encyclopaedia Britannica Inc.)

6. Lodwick, G.S. (1971). *The Bones and Joints*. (Chicago: Year Book Medical Publishers)

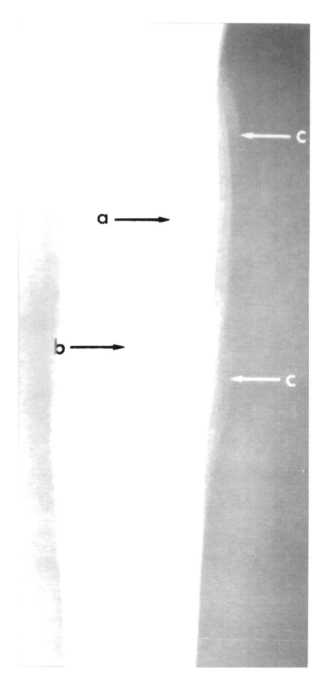

Figure 1. 'The five layers of periosteal new bone produce the classic onion-peel appearance.' Reprinted from *The Bones and Joints* by Lodwick (1971)[5], published by Year Book Medical Publishers, Chicago. Copyright 1971 with ACR. Reprinted with permission

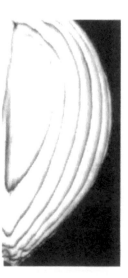

Figure 2. A large red onion

PARCHMENT HEART

Sir William Osler[1] introduced this term in the sixth edition (1905) of his book, *The Principles and Practice of Medicine*. He described 'an extraordinary heart in the McGill College Museum showing a parchment-like thinning of the walls with uniform dilatation of all the chambers; in places in the right auricle and ventricle, only the epicardium remains.' Drawings of the heart that Osler described were printed in a 1950 article[2] (Figure 1). At that time no other similar case was found in a search of the literature. In 1952, two similar cases were reported. The first, reported as the weekly clinicopathological exercise in the May 15 issue of the *New England Journal of Medicine*, was a 24-year-old woman with extreme thinning of the right ventricle and right auricle[3]. Although the Osler case was mentioned in the discussion of this patient's case the final diagnosis given was 'cardiac dilatation of the right heart, extreme, ? congenital.' The second case, reported by Henry Uhl (Johns Hopkins) concerned an 8-month-old infant who died of complications of a congenital heart disorder[4]. At autopsy, almost total absence of the myocardium was noted exclusively in the right ventricular wall and the auricle (atrium) was hypertrophied. Uhl did not mention Osler's description. Uhl's name is now used as the eponym for this disorder which radiologists can diagnose by angiography, echocardiography, computerized tomography or magnetic resonance imaging (Figure 2).

Parchment is 'a sheet-like material made from animal skin.' King Eumenes II's library at Pergamum in Asia Minor 'is traditionally regarded as the place where parchment [Figure 3] ... is said to have been invented. The source of this tradition is Pliny's Natural History: when owing to the rivalry between King Ptolemy and King Eumenes about their libraries, Ptolemy suppressed the export of papyrus, parchment was invented at Pergamum and afterwards the employment of the material on which the immortality of human beings depends, spread indiscriminately.'[5]

References

1. Osler, W. (1905). *The Principles and Practice of Medicine*, 6th edn, p. 820 (New York: D. Appleton & Co.)

2. Segall, H.N. (1950). Parchment heart (Osler). *Am. Heart J.*, 40, 948–50

3. Castleman, B. and Towne, V.W. (1952). Case 38201. *N. Engl. J. Med.*, 246, 785–90

4. Uhl, H.S.M. (1952). A previously undescribed congenital malformation of the heart: almost total absence of the myocardium of the right ventricle. *Bull. Johns Hopkins Hosp.*, 91, 197–205

5. Reed, R. (1975). *The Nature and Making of Parchment*, pp. 3–7. (Leeds: Elmete Press)

6. Bewick, D. J., Chandler, B. M. and Montague, T. J. (1986). Dilated right ventricular cardiomyopathy. *Chest*, 90, 300–2

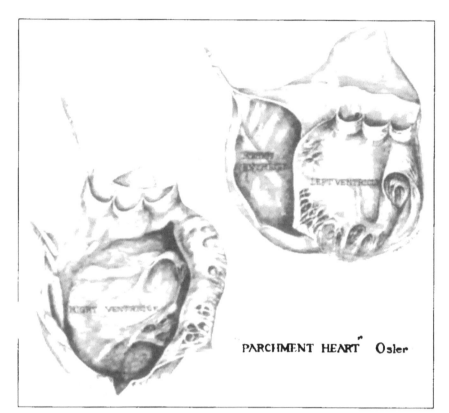

PARCHMENT HEART Osler

Figure 1. 'Two views of the heart with walls of parchment-like thinness.' Reprinted from Segall[2]. Parchment heart (Osler). *Am. Heart J.*, 1950, **40**, 948–50, with permission of Mosby-Yearbook Inc.

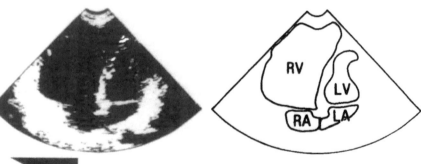

Figure 2. Parchment heart shown in stop-frame four-chamber real-time echocardiogram (left) and diagnostic sketch (right) illustrating the large right ventricle. Reprinted from Bewick *et al.*[6]. Dilated right ventricular cardiomyopathy. *Chest*, 1986, **90**, 300–2, with permission

Figure 3. Sheepskin (parchment) diploma

PHRYGIAN CAP GALLBLADDER

Phrygian cap gallbladders are those with a 'folded fundus.' This anatomic peculiarity was described by Julius Bartel[1] (Wien University) in 1918. He was a pathologist who had noted the varied appearance of the gallbladder fundus in autopsy specimens. The fundus in some cases was 'bent down ... after the manner of a Phrygian cap' (Figure 1). He considered the various fold patterns to be the result of a developmental abnormality. This anomaly used to be seen by radiologists on oral cholecystograms. It is still occasionally demonstrated during ultrasound or computerized tomographic examinations of the abdomen.

Evarts Graham and Warren Cole (Washington University, St Louis) developed the technique of intravenous cholecystography in the early 1920s[2]. Oral cholecystography (OCG) followed in 1925[3]. The OCG was a popular and useful test for gallbladder disease until it was superseded by radioisotope scans and ultrasound examinations in the 1980s. Today intravenous and oral cholecystography are procedures rarely done in the United States.

The Phrygians dominated Asia Minor between the twelfth and seventh centuries BC. One of their rulers was the legendary king Midas. These people were later valued as slaves by the Greeks. The Phrygian cap, a soft felt or wool, conical head-dress with a pointed crown that curls forward, was 'worn by emancipated slaves as a symbol of their freedom'[4] (Figure 2).

References

1. Bartel, J. (1918). Ueber eine Formanomalie der Gallenblase und ihre biologischen Beziehungen. *Wien Klin. Wochenschr.*, 31, 605–11

2. Cole, W.H. (1960). The story of cholecystography. *Am. J. Surg.*, 99, 206–21

3. Whitaker, L.R., Milliken, G. and Vogt, E.C. (1925). The oral administration of sodium tetraiodophenolphthalein for cholecystography. *Surg. Gynecol. Obstet.*, 40, 847–51

4. Phrygian cap. In *The New Encyclopaedia Britannica*, 1990, 15th edn, Vol. 9, p. 408. (Chicago: Encyclopaedia Britannica Inc.)

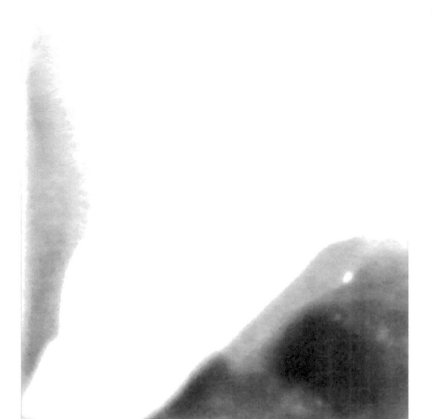

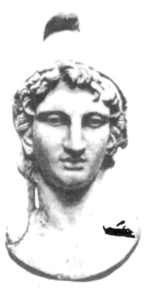

Figure 1. Cholecystogram showing Phrygian cap appearance. Case from University of Maryland teaching file

Figure 2. Youth wearing a Phrygian cap, Roman copy of a Greek original

PICKET-FENCE AND STACK OF COINS SIGNS

The picket-fence sign, in radiologic terminology, is the spiked appearance of intestinal mucosal folds seen in some cases of intramural hemorrhage by barium examination. Jerome Wiot and colleagues[1] (University of Cincinnati) described this sign in a 1961 report that described the roentgenologic picture of two patients who had duodenal hematomas induced by coumarin. They said, 'The normal feathery appearance was lost and the duodenal margins showed 'spikes' of varying height. Longitudinal folds were not visible, so the mucosal pattern had a 'picket-fence' appearance' (Figure 1). This pattern can be seen elsewhere in the small and large intestine as was reported in a 1964 review of intramural intestinal bleeding. In the jejunum and ileum, Khilnani and co-workers[2] (Mount Sinai Hospital, New York) used the stack of coins imagery (Figure 2) to describe its appearance. 'The small intestine fold pattern may have a highly characteristic appearance and varies slightly with the different entities producing intramural hemorrhage. There is uniform, regular thickening of the folds, sharp delineation of their margins, and a parallel arrangement producing a symmetric spike-like configuration simulating a stack of coins.'[2] Other processes, besides hemorrhage, may lead to thickening of the bowel wall with a similar appearance (e.g. edema, cellular infiltration) and they should be considered in the differential diagnosis.

A picket is defined as a 'pointed stake, post, or peg, driven into the ground; used for various purposes, [for example] ... the construction of a stockade or fence'[3] (Figure 3).

'True coinage began soon after 650 BC. The sixth century Greek poet Xenophanes, quoted by the historian Herodotus, ascribed its invention to the Lydians, 'the first to strike and use coins of gold and silver.''[4] Figure 4 shows a stack of coins.

References

1. Wiot, J.F., Weinstein, A.S. and Felson, B. (1961). Duodenal hematoma induced by coumarin. *Am. J. Roentgenol.*, 86, 70–5

2. Khilnani, M.T., Marshak, R.H., Eliasoph, J. and Wolf, B.S. (1964). Intramural intestinal hemorrhage. *Am. J. Roentgenol.*, 92, 1061–71

3. Simpson, J. and Weiner, E. (eds.) (1989). *Oxford English Dictionary*, 2nd edn, Vol. 11, p. 773. (Oxford: Clarendon Press)

4. Coins and coinage. In *The New Encyclopaedia Britannica*, 1990, 15th edn, Vol. 16, pp. 529–55. (Chicago: Encyclopaedia Britannica Inc.)

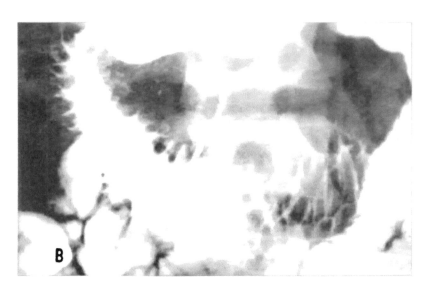

Figure 1. 'There are marked mucosal changes of the duodenum, with rigid thickened folds and narrow troughs between them. The pattern simulates a 'picket-fence'.' Reprinted from Wiot et al.[1]. Duodenal hematoma induced by coumarin. *Am. J. Roentgenol.*, 1961, **86**, 70–5, with the permission of the ARRS

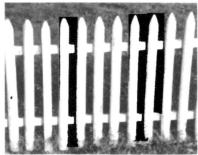

Figure 3. A picket fence

Figure 2. 'Idiopathic thrombocytopenic purpura with hemorrhage into the small intestinal wall. The folds in the distal ileum are thickened and have a stacked coin appearance.' Reprinted from Khilnani et al.[2]. Intramural intestinal haemorrhage. *Am. J. Roentgenol.*, 1964, **92**, 1061–71, with the permission of the ARRS

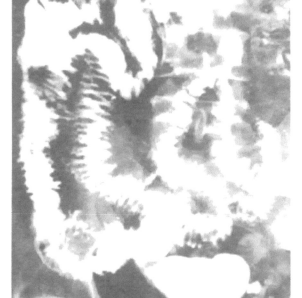

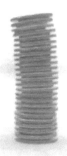

Figure 4. A coin stack

PICTURE FRAME SIGN

'One picture is worth more than a thousand words' says the Chinese proverb[1]. Picture frames can also be very expressive, as is the case with the term used for one type of Pagetoid change seen in a vertebral body. Georg Schmorl[2,3] (1861–1932), who wrote extensively on disorders of the spine, gave radiologists this picture-frame analogy in two of his articles that dealt with Pagetoid changes in the spine. He correlated the gross pathologic and roentgenographic changes of Paget's disease in the spinal column. Schmorl found that in Paget's disease the trabeculae at the edges of the vertebral bodies seemed compacted and were more dense than those in the midbody. To him, these compact dense trabeculae surrounding the midbody suggested the likeness of a framework or picture frame (rahmenartig). This appearance of a coarsened thickened framework, outlining a vertebral body, is a roentgen classic that is diagnostic of Paget's disease (Figures 1 and 2). No other words are necessary when one sees this 'picture frame'.

'The picture frame, as it exists today, is derived from the doorway or entrance to temples, palaces and cathedrals ... the importance of the door framing an impressive picture of the interior was never overlooked. The earliest examples of [picture] frame-like decorations or borders bear a great resemblance to door frames'[4] and 'date from the Middle Ages.'[5] Figure 3 shows a framed picture of Sir James Paget.

References

1. Bartlett, J. (ed.) (1980). Chinese proverb. In *Familiar Quotations*, 15th edn, p. 132. (Boston: Little, Brown and Company)

2. Schmorl, G. (1927). Ueber die an den wirbelbandscheiben vorkommenden Ausdehnungs – und Zerreissungsvorgänge und die dadurch an ihnen und der Wirbelspongiosa hervorgerufenen veränderungen. *Verh. Dtsche. Pathol. Ges.*, 22, 250–62

3. Schmorl, G. (1932). Über Ostitis deformans Paget. *Virchows Arch. Pathol. Anat. Physiol. Klin. Med.*, 283, 694–751

4. Landon, E. (1945). *Picture Framing*, p. 1. (New York: American Artists Group Inc.)

5. Burns, J.T. (1978). *Framing Pictures*, p. 11 (New York: Charles Scribner's Sons)

6. Paget, J. and Paget, S. (1902). *Memoirs and Letters of Sir James Paget*. (London: Longman's Green and Company)

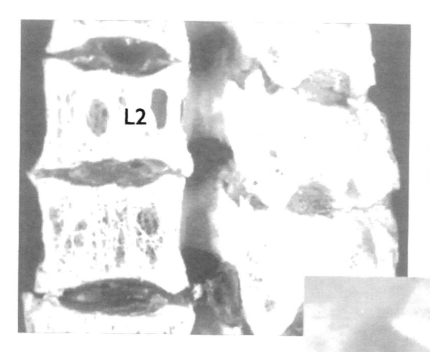

Figure 1. Photograph of specimen from Schmorl's work clearly showing the framework phenomenon in the second lumbar vertebra (L2). Reprinted from Schmorl[3]. Über Ostitis deformans Paget. *Virchows Arch. Pathol. Anat. Physiol. Klin. Med.*, 1932, **283**, 694–751, with permission of Springer-Verlag

Figure 2. Lateral spine radiograph with typical picture-frame appearance due to Paget's disease. Case courtesy of Dr C. Resnik, University of Maryland

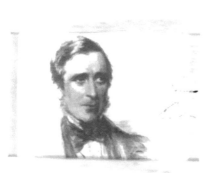

Figure 3. Framed picture of Sir James Paget (retouched). From *Memoirs and Letters of Sir James Paget*. By Paget and Paget (1902)[4], published by Longman's Green and Company, London

PINE TREE (CHRISTMAS TREE) BLADDER

Charles Ney and John Duff[1] reviewed the cysto-urethrogram findings of the neuogenic bladder, in a 1950 article, 'because of the great resurgence of interest in the neurogenic bladder as a result of [World War II] injuries.' One of the findings they discussed was the pine tree shaped bladder, 'a descriptive term applied to bladders which taper towards the dome, and associated usually with trabeculation and often with cellule formation and sacculation. Such a silhouette gives the entire structure the appearance of a pine tree. This type of bladder can be either hyper- or hypotonic in type. It is for the most part characteristic of neuro-genic bladder'[1] (Figure 1). Other terms used to describe this appearance of the bladder include pine cone and Christmas tree.

Pine trees are found in the genus *Pinus*, a subset of the conifers, class Coniferopsida (Figure 2). 'The coniferophytes are the most varied gymnosperms. The world's oldest trees are the 4900-year-old bristlecone pines ... The largest trees are the giant sequoias ... the very tallest are the redwoods ... Conifers provide all the world's softwood timber ... and about 45 percent of the world's annual lumber production ... Conifers appeared first toward the end of the Late Carboniferous epoch (320 to 286 million years ago).'[2]

The modern Christmas tree originated in western Germany. The main prop of a popular medieval play about Adam and Eve was a fir tree hung with apples (paradise tree). The Germans set up a paradise tree in their homes on December 24, the religious feast day of Adam and Eve[3].

References

1. Ney, C. and Duff, J. (1950). Cysto-urethrography: its role in diagnosis of neurogenic bladder. *J. Urol.*, 63, 640–52

2. Gymnosperms. In *The New Encyclopaedia Britannica*, 1990, 15th edn, Vol. 20, pp. 451–3. (Chicago: Encyclopaedia Britannica Inc.)

3. Christmas tree. In *The New Encyclopaedia Britannica*, 1990, 15th edn, Vol. 3, p. 284. (Chicago: Encyclopaedia Britannica Inc.)

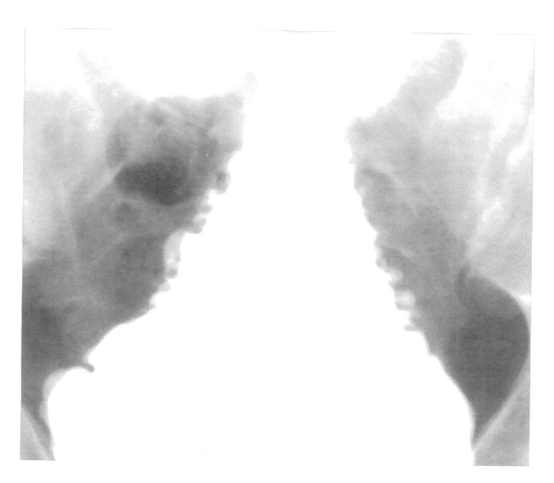

Figure 1. Radiograph of contrast-filled 'pine tree' bladder (author's case)

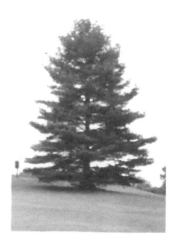

Figure 2. A pine tree

PLAYBOY BUNNY SIGN

The Playboy bunny sign is one of the few classic radiologic signs in use that did not appear originally in the medical literature. Perhaps more appropriately, it was initially described in a letter to the editor of *Playboy* magazine[1]. Anatomically, as seen during an ultrasound examination of the liver, it represents the confluence of the hepatic veins with the inferior vena cava: the head of the bunny being the inferior vena cava and the ears the hepatic veins[2] (Figure 1). The original patient reportedly had mild congestive heart failure that made the veins more prominent than usual (Joseph Dils, personal communication). This sign is used to recognize the intersection of these important vascular structures. One can then more precisely localize any abnormality detected in the liver. Precise localization of primary and metastatic liver lesions is very important in this age of aggressive treatment with intra-arterial chemotherapy and subtotal surgical resection.

Arthur Paul, a 28-year-old Chicago freelance designer and graduate of the Chicago Institute of Design, drew the Playboy rabbit symbol (Figure 2) as the logo for Hugh Hefner's new magazine in 1953. Hefner himself decided to use the rabbit (after the original stag idea was discarded) since it 'is a playboy of the animal world, noted for both its playfulness and its sexual prowess.'[3]

References

1. Dils, J.P. (1979). Rabbit Test. *Playboy*, Jan., 28

2. Bartrum, R.J. and Crow, H.C. (1983). *Real-time Ultrasound*, pp. 78–9. (Philadelphia: W.B. Saunders Co.)

3. Hefner, H.M. (1994). Golden Dreams. *Playboy*, Jan., 114–272

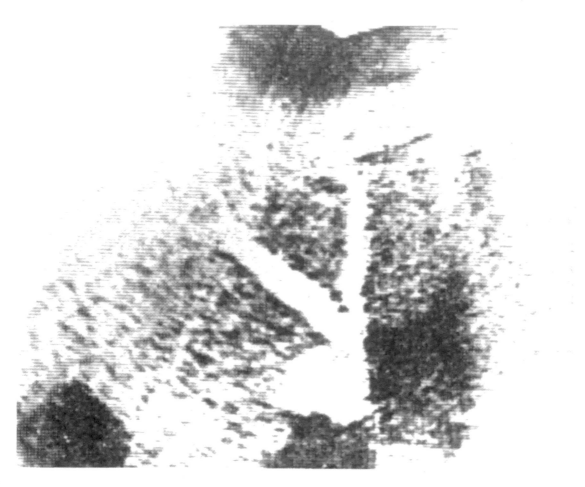

Figure 1. 'Ultrasound study of a human liver.'
Reprinted from Dils'. Rabbit test. *Playboy*, 1979, with
permission of Playboy Enterprises Inc. (PEI)

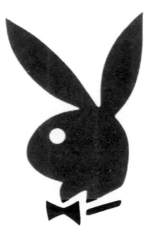

Figure 2. Playboy's rabbit.
Courtesy of Playboy Enterprises Inc. (PEI)

PORCELAIN GALLBLADDER

The term 'porzellangallenblase' (porcelain gall-bladder) was proposed by Heinrich Flörcken[1] (Frankfurt), in 1929, to denote the changes seen in an inflammatory condition that caused calcification of the gallbladder wall. It was presumably meant to emphasize 'the brittle consistency and bluish discoloration of the wall'[2]. Although Flörcken considered it to be the result of a previous inflammatory process and of no consequence, other cases were soon reported that disputed its supposed innocuous nature[3]. These gallbladders may function poorly and often contain gallstones. Gallbladder carcinoma, a relatively uncommon gastrointestinal tract malignancy, has an increased incidence in cases of porcelain gallbladder. The pattern of calcification in the gallbladder wall is important when one is considering the possibility of carcinoma (Figure 1). 'Incomplete calcification of the wall is much more likely to be associated with [gallbladder carcinoma] than the complete type.'[4] This is likely to be due to the fact that with complete calcification the mucosal epithelium is totally replaced by dense connective tissue that is not prone to undergo a cancerous change. Ultrasound and computerized tomography can also be used to detect and evaluate porcelain gallbladders. A giant gallstone is one plain film mimic that also has been reported to have an association with the development of a gallbladder carcinoma.

'Porcelain [and] china are synonymous as true porcelain was found and developed in China and ... it was porcelain to which Europeans referred when they used the term china. It is made of fusible silicates of alumina (called petuntse) and nonfusible silicates of alumina (called kaolin)'[5] (Figure 2).

References

1. Flörcken, H. (1929). Die 'porzellangallenblase' (chole-cystopathia chronica calcarea). Dtsche. Z. Chir., 216, 264–70

2. Berk, R.N., Armbuster, T.G. and Saltzstein, S.L. (1973). Carcinoma in the porcelain gallbladder. Radiology, 106, 29–31 (Attributed in this article, and others, to Osler, W. (1925). Principles and Practice of Medicine, 10th edn, but not found there or in any later edition of this work)

3. Goldhamer, K. (1930). Über petrifikation der Gallen-blasenwandung. Fortschr. Geb. Rontgensrt., 42, 95–102

4. Daly, B.D., Cheung, H., Arnold, M. and Metreweli, C. (1993). Ultrasound in the diagnosis of gall-bladder carcinoma in Chinese patients. Clin. Radiol., 48, 41–4

5. Cox, W.E. (1944). The Book of Pottery and Porcelain, p. xv. (New York: Crown Publishers)

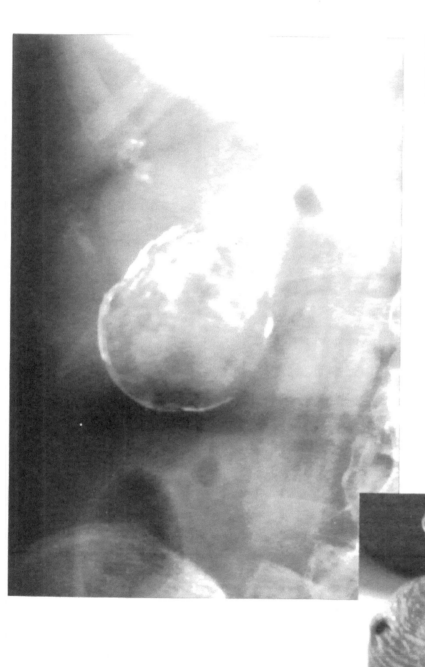

Figure 1. Abdominal
radiograph showing calcified
gallbladder. Case courtesy
of Dr D. Fleming, Bethesda
Naval Hospital

Figure 2. Porcellaneous jug, third
century AD Field Mus., Chicago

PRUNED TREE AND LEAFLESS TREE SIGNS

In a 1951 review of the causes of pulmonary hypertension, William Evans[1] described the pathologic and radiologic features of emphysema in a series of patients. Postmortem pulmonary arteriograms showed 'pruning of the terminal branches of the pulmonary tree giving it an appearance of a denuded shrub in winter contrasting with the leafy bush in spring which typifies the healthy pulmonary circulation'[1] (Figure 1). Microscopically these abrupt pulmonary vascular terminations were said to be due to 'endarteritis fibrosa.' These findings in the living patient meant impending heart failure and an 'unfavorable outlook.' Evans used the word 'pruning' in the accompanying figure legend. The pruned tree terminology is more commonly used now than the phrase 'denuded shrub.'

This angiographic finding described by Evans has also been applied to plain chest radiographs. It is now used to describe the findings of pulmonary artery hypertension from any cause. Evans[1] said, 'It is opined here that the same mechanism is operating in most examples of gross pulmonary hypertension.' The pruned-tree sign should not be confused with the bronchographic 'leafless-tree' sign of bronchioloalveolar cell carcinoma[2].

Pruning, for the horticulturist, is the act of trimming branches either to stimulate new growth or to remove diseased or unproductive limbs. It is said to be 'one of the most important operations connected with the management of trees'[3] (Figure 2). The human pulmonary tree is not only pruned by disease processes, it may prune itself. This happens whenever pulmonary bloodflow is directed away from poorly aerated areas of the lung and is readily shown on radionuclide ventilation/perfusion scans.

References

1. Evans, W. (1951). Congenital pulmonary hypertension. *Proc. R. Soc. Med.*, 44, 600–8

2. Zheutlin, N., Lasser, E.C. and Rigler, L.G. (1954). Bronchographic abnormalities in alveolar cell carcinoma of the lung. *Dis. Chest*, 25, 542–49

3. Barry, P. (1863). *The Fruit Garden; A Treatise*, p. 83. (Rochester, NY)

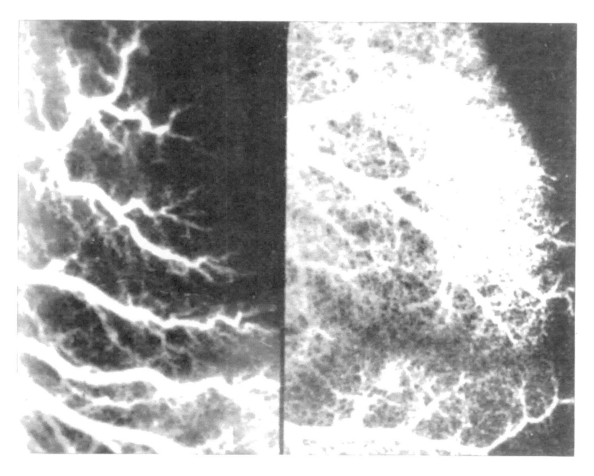

Figure 1. 'Emphysema. Pulmonary arteriogram showing pruning effect of terminal branches in patient with pulmonary hypertension and heart failure [left], and compared with normal control [right].' Reprinted from Evans[1]. Congenital pulmonary hypertension. *Proc. R. Soc. Med.*, 1951, **44**, 600–8, with permission of the Royal Society of Medicine

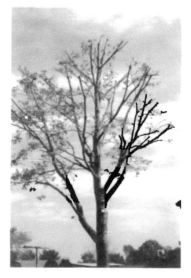

Figure 2. A pruned tree

RIBBON (TWISTED-RIBBON) RIBS

In their 1948 discussion of the radiologic features of neurofibromatosis, John Holt and Edwin Wright[1] (University of Michigan) emphasized the rib changes that could simulate the rib notching seen in patients with coarctation of the aorta. They studied 127 patients, with von Recklinghausen's neurofibromatosis, seen during a 13-year period. Credit is given to earlier authors who had described pressure defects[2], and pits or caves in the ribs[3]. However, it was Holt and Wright who used the 'twisted-ribbon' analogy to describe the now classic appearance of the rib abnormalities in neurofibromatosis (Figure 1). They recognized that 'There probably is nothing precisely characteristic about this type of rib erosion, but as it is so infrequently associated with intrathoracic tumors other than neurofibromata, it must be regarded as having considerable diagnostic significance.' The twisted-ribbon term appears in the figure legends that accompany the article's illustrations.

Hooshang Taybi[4] in his book, *Radiology of Syndromes, Metabolic Disorders, and Skeletal Dysplasias,* listed achondrogenesis, trisomies and osteogenesis imperfecta among the disorders to consider in the differential diagnosis when one encounters twisted or ribbon ribs.

A ribbon is a 'narrow woven band of some fine material, as silk or satin, used to ornament clothing or headgear, or utilized for other purposes.'[5] Ribbons have been used in this way since at least the fifteenth century (Figure 2).

References

1. Holt, J.F. and Wright, E.M. (1948). The radiologic features of neurofibromatosis. *Radiology,* 51, 647–63

2. Stahnke, E. (1992). Über Knochenveränderungen bei Neurofibromatose. *Dtsche. Z. Chir.,* 168, 6–18

3. Norgaard, F. (1937). Osseous changes in Recklinghausen's neurofibromatosis. *Acta Radiol.,* 18, 460–70

4. Taybi, H. (1990). *Radiology of Syndromes, Metabolic Diseases, and Skeletal Dysplasias,* 3rd edn., p. 882. (Chicago: Year Book Medical Publishers)

5 Simpson, J. and Weiner, E. In *Oxford English Dictionary,* 1989, 2nd edn., Vol. 13, pp. 882–4. (Oxford: Clarendon Press)

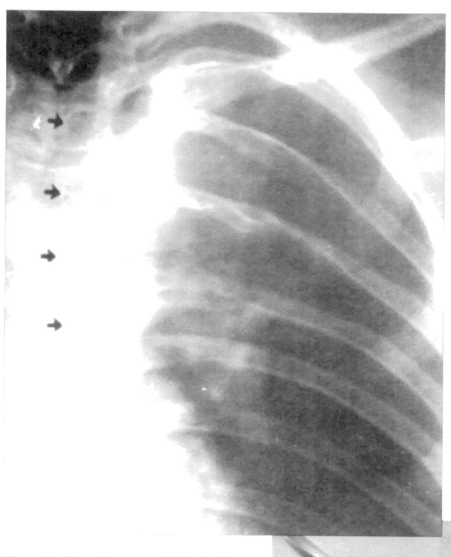

Figure 1. 'Extensive erosion of left side of upper thoracic spine and adjoining ribs due to neurofibroma arising within the spinal canal and extending into the thorax. Note the twisted-ribbon appearance of the fourth and fifth ribs.' Reprinted from Holt and Wright[1]. The radiologic features of neurofibromatosis. *Radiology*, 1948, 51, 647–63, with permission of the RSNA

Figure 2. A twisted ribbon

RUGGER-JERSEY SPINE

C.E. Dent (University College Hospital, London), in an invited commentary on a 1955 case report of secondary hyperparathyroidism by S. Karani, in the *Proceedings of the Royal Society of Medicine*, said of the patient's X-rays, 'the vertebral bodies are more dense in the upper and lower parts than in their middle thus showing the appearance of horizontal striations which Dr Hodson and I are beginning to call the 'rugger-jersey' sign'[1] (Figure 1). The pattern was apparently reminiscent of the alternating colored 'hoops' on a rugby player's jersey, a design that was popular at the time (Figure 2). Dent was a co-author of another earlier paper that discussed osteosclerotic findings in patients with chronic renal failure[2]. Three cases were discussed. Two of the patients had 'rugger-jersey' spine changes described, although the term was not used in that article. Dent and Hodson[3] also published a review article in 1954 of radiologic changes in metabolic disorders that also showed their leading role in this subject area.

The sclerotic changes leading to the rugger-jersey pattern were not well understood at the time. Dent said, 'We have no serious suggestions to make as to the mechanism for the formation of this osteosclerosis.'[1] Indeed, the exact cause of the osteosclerosis is still not known.

'A tablet set in the ivy-covered wall at Rugby ... reads, 'This stone commemorates the exploit of William Webb Ellis who with a fine disregard for the rules of football [soccer] as played in his time first took the ball in his arms and ran with it thus originating the distinctive feature of the Rugby game AD 1823.' '[4]

References

1. Karani, S. (1955). Secondary hyperparathyroidism. Primary renal failure. *Proc. R. Soc. Med.*, **48**, 527–30, with comment by C.E. Dent

2. Crawford, T., Dent, C.E., Lucas, P., Martin, N.H. and Nassim, J.R. (1954). Osteosclerosis associated with chronic renal failure. *Lancet*, ii, 981–8

3. Dent, C.E. and Hodson, C.J. (1954). Radiological changes associated with certain metabolic bone diseases. *Br. J. Radiol.*, **27**, 605–18

4. Weyand, A.M. (1955). *The Saga of American Football*, p. 9. (New York: The Macmillan Co.)

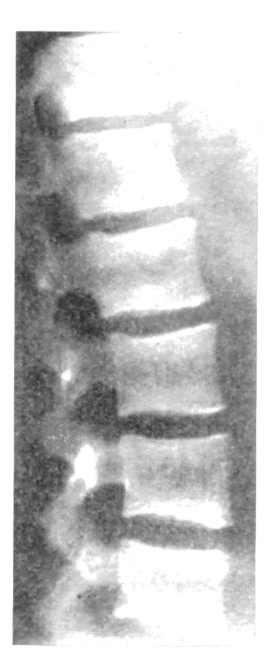

Figure 1. 'Lumbar spine of case 2, showing increased density of upper and lower parts of each vertebral body.' Reprinted from Crawford et al.[2] Osteosclerosis associated with chronic renal failure. *Lancet*, 1954, ii, 981–988, with permission of The Lancet Ltd

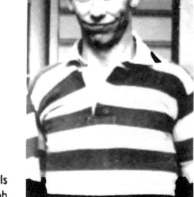

Figure 2. 'Hooped' rugger jersey of Rolls Royce Rugby Club 1950–51. Photograph courtesy of Dr K.J. Fairbairn, Derby, UK

'S' (GOLDEN'S) SIGN

One of the fundamental radiographic signs of a bronchogenic carcinoma is postobstructive atelectasis. Ross Golden[1] (Presbyterian Hospital, Columbia) reported five such cases at the Twenty-fifth Annual Meeting of the American Roentgen Ray Society, held in Swampscott, Massachusetts in 1924. Two of the cases involved the right upper lobe and showed the now classic sigmoid curvature of the minor fissure – the Golden 'S' sign (Figure 1). This sign is produced by the double curve of the minor fissure – concave laterally but convex medially where it bends around the tumor mass in the hilum. The medial convexity indicates that there is a mass lesion causing the upper lobe volume loss. Golden[1] himself did not use the 'S' terminology in his subsequent article. Perhaps the meeting's setting in serene Swampscott suggested the 'S' symbolism (Figure 2).

Golden did not consider atelectasis to be solely characteristic of bronchial carcinomas since he recognized that it 'may be produced by any process which occludes a bronchus.'[1] He introduced his paper by saying, 'The problem of the diagnosis of primary neoplasm of the lung seems at the present time to be attracting considerable attention, if one may judge by the frequency with which the subject is discussed at medical meetings.'[1] (How little has changed in 70 years.) His objective was 'to point out the remarkable changes in the shadows on the roentgenogram which may take place as the disease progresses and to indicate the role which broncho-stenosis plays in the production of these changes.'[1] He concluded with some time-honored wisdom for us all, 'It is obvious that a correlation of clinical and laboratory information is necessary in order to reach a definite conclusion in these somewhat confusing cases. But when these shadows occupying the position of one or more lobes present themselves for consideration, if the possibility of bronchostenosis due to neoplasm is mentioned, the diagnostic machine will at least be started on the right road.'[1]

'[W]e can date the origin of the alphabet, in the second quarter of the second millennium BC, which is now commonly dated 1730–1580 BC. All the other more important attempts at alphabetic writing ... can also be attributed to the period. Both the conception of consonantal writing and the acrophonic principle may have been borrowed from Egypt. But only the Syro-Palestinian Semites ... created the alphabetic writing, from which have descended all past and present alphabets. [T]he Latin alphabet was borrowed from the Etruscan in the very early stage of this latter alphabet. The creation of the Latin alphabet may be dated in the seventh century BC. Of the three Etruscan s-sounds, the Romans retained the Greek sigma.'[2]

References
1. Golden, R. (1925). The effect of bronchostenosis upon the roentgen-ray shadows in carcinoma of the bronchus. *Am. J. Roentgenol.*, 13, 21–30

2. Diringer, D. (1948). *The Alphabet - A Key to the History of Mankind*, pp. 214–534. (New York: Philosophical Library Inc.)

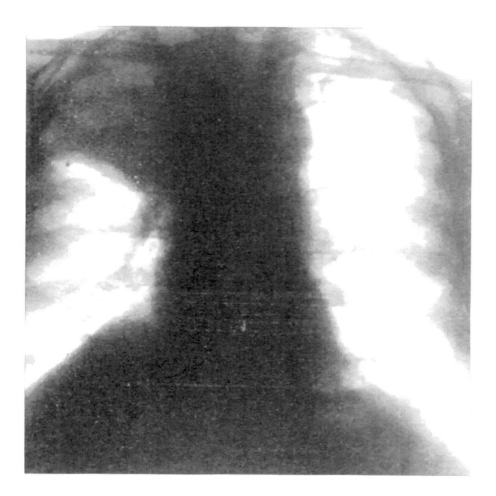

Figure 1. 'The area of the right upper lobe is
occupied by a dense shadow with a sharply defined
concave lower margin.' Reprinted from Golden[1].
The effect of bronchosterosis upon the roentgen-
ray shadow in carcinoma of the bronchus. *Am. J.
Roentgenol.*, 1925, **13**, 21–30, with permission of the
ARRS

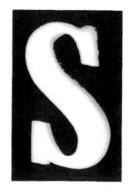

Figure 2. A golden 'S'

SABER-SHEATH TRACHEA

Saber-sheath trachea is the term for the narrow bowed tracheal air column seen on chest radiographs (Figure 1) of patients with chronic obstructive pulmonary disease (COPD). It was Reginald Greene and Gerhard Lechner[1] who first associated this tracheal abnormality with patients who had altered pulmonary function. The term, alterssabelscheidentrachea (saber-sheath trachea), had previously been used by pathologists who seem to have regarded it as a normal consequence of aging[2]. Greene and Lechner presented data from 13 patients seen at the Massachusetts General Hospital. The coronal diameter of the intrathoracic trachea in each patient was one-half or less that of the corresponding sagittal diameter. On frontal and lateral chest radiographs, this finding allows the radiologist to suggest the diagnosis of COPD. Clinical information and pulmonary function data supported the diagnosis of COPD in Greene and Lechner's cases. Recognition of the saber-sheath abnormality as a sign of COPD has been emphasized since tracheal compression or distortion in other planes may be indicative of a mediastinal mass.

Sabers (with sheaths) are a type of cavalry sword with a curved blade specially adapted for cutting[3] (Figure 2). They were introduced to western armies from the Orient in the eighteenth century[4].

References

1. Greene, R. and Lechner, G.L. (1975). 'Saber-Sheath' trachea: a clinical and functional study of marked coronal narrowing of the intrathoracic trachea. *Radiology*, 115, 265–8

2. Simmonds, M. (1905). Über Alterssäbelscheidentrachea. *Virchows Arch. Pathol. Anat. Physiol. Klin. Med.*, 179, 15–28

3. Sabre. In Simpson, J. and Weiner, E. (eds.) *Oxford English Dictionary*, 1989, 2nd edn., Vol. 14, p. 324. (Oxford: Clarendon Press)

4. Sabre. In *The New Encyclopaedia Britannica*, 1990, 15th edn., Vol. 10, p. 283. (Chicago: Encyclopaedia Britannica Inc.)

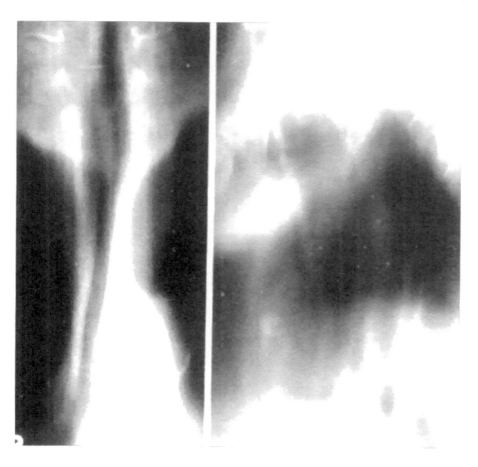

Figure 1. Saber-sheath trachea seen in 'anteroposterior (left) and lateral tomographic sections (right) through the intrathoracic trachea. Note the abrupt change from marked coronal narrowing to a more rounded shape at the thoracic outlet.' Reprinted from Greene and Lechner[1]. 'Saber-Sheath' trachea: a clinical and functional study of marked coronal narrowing of the intrathoracic trachea. *Radiology*, 1975, **115**, 265–268, with permission of the RSNA

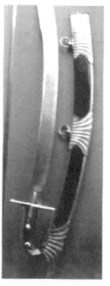

Figure 2. Saber and sheath on exhibit at Musée de l'Armée, Paris

SABRE SHIN

French disease was one of the early favorite terms for the illness later known as syphilis. French armies were blamed for spreading the disease throughout Europe during wars in the late fifteenth century. Each European country in turn seems to have blamed another for the disease. Thus, it was also known as Spanish disease, Italian disease, etc. 'The Verona physician, Girolamo Fracastoro (1483–1553) named the disease 'syphilis' in his 1530 poem, *Syphilis sive Morbus Gallicus*, that described the plight of an afflicted shepherd.'[1]

One of the manifestations of hereditary syphilis is the characteristic sabre-shin deformity (Figure 1). The term *'tibia en lame de sabre'* was used by Alfred Fournier[2] (1832–1914) in his book on hereditary syphilis written in 1886. In the chapter on osseous deformities, he discussed the pseudo-rachitic curvature of the tibia. He recognized this as an 'important diagnostic sign of hereditary syphilis' and considered the deformity to be nearly pathognomonic. Although we know that this deformity, due to the chronic syphilitic osteomyelitis, can be seen with other treponemal infections (e.g. yaws) and certain other chronic infections, it will always be classically associated with syphilis by most radiologists.

'A sabre (saber) is a heavy military sword with a long cutting edge (Figure 2) and, often, a curved blade, derived from a Hungarian cavalry sword introduced from the Orient in the 18th century.'[3]

References

1. Bynum, W.F. and Porter, R. (eds.) *Companion Encyclopedia of the History of Medicine*, 1993, p. 564. (London: Routledge)

2. Fournier, A. (1886). *La Syphilis Héréditaire Tardive*, pp. 47–9. (Paris: G. Mason)

3. Sabre. In *The New Encyclopaedia Britannica*, 1990, 15th edn., Vol. 10, p. 283. (Chicago: Encyclopaedia Britannica Inc.)

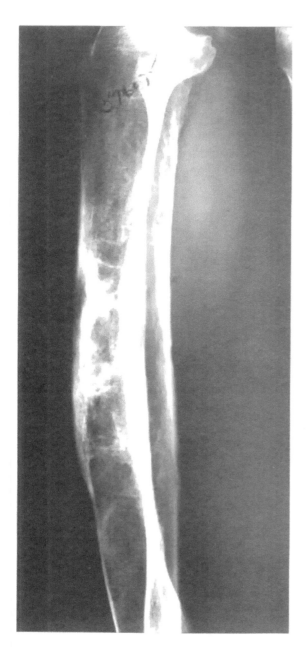

Figure 1. Lateral radiograph of syphilitic tibia showing sabre-shin deformity. Case courtesy of the Armed Forces Institute of Pathology

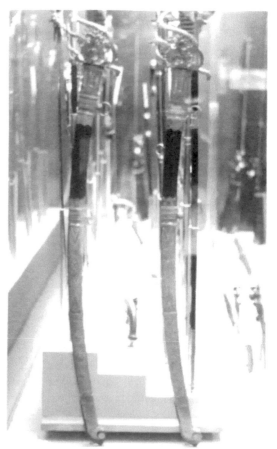

Figure 2. Sabers on exhibit at Musée de l'Armée, Paris

SAIL AND SPINNAKER SAIL SIGNS

'There are numerous variations in structure and function, in posture and in the position of organs, which fall within natural limits, but have nevertheless been frequently misinterpreted as pathological findings.' These words introduce the 1948 article by Kemp and colleagues[1] that pointed out a sail-like appearance of the normal thymus (Figures 1 and 2). 'The radiographs of a number of young children, in the Child Health Survey conducted by the Institute of Social Medicine at Oxford, show a sail-like triangular opacity projecting from the mediastinum, which investigation has proved to be the thymus gland.'[1] The sail sign was seen in 44 (8.8%) of 498 children examined at 6 months of age. None had pulmonary or cardiac symptoms. Three cases had autopsy proof. The authors credit Sir James Brailsford for being the first to suggest 'that this shadow was the thymus.'

John Moseley[2] (Mount Sinai Hospital, New York), in 1960, added the 'spinnaker sail' sign to our lexicon. This sign in contrast with the normal sail sign described above represents a loculated pneumomediastinum with displacement of the thymic lobe (Figure 3). Moseley said, 'the crescentic configuration of the thymic lobe, in this situation, is similar to that of a wind-blown spinnaker sail' (Figure 4).

'There are no records of the early beginnings of naval architecture ... because man's ability to build primitive vessels goes considerably further back in time than the art of recording human knowledge and experience. [A]round 4000 BC, an Egyptian artist painted a vessel which clearly shows a square sail set on one mast. [C]irca 3000 BC the Egyptians were navigating the Nile in strong, serviceable sailing boats.'[3]

The spinnaker sail was developed in the 1860s. The crew of the yacht Sphinx christened their new 'sail a 'spinxer,' and this name was gradually changed to 'spinnaker' as we know it today.'[3]

References

1. Kemp, F.H., Morley, H.M.C. and Emrys-Roberts, E. (1948). A sail-like triangular projection from the mediastinum: a radiographic appearance of the thymus gland. Br. J. Radiol., 21, 618–24

2. Moseley, J.E. (1960). Loculated pneumomediastinum in the newborn – a thymic 'spinnaker sail' sign. Radiology, 75, 788–90

3. Baader, J. (1979). The Sailing Yacht, pp. 8–157. (New York: W.W. Norton and Co. Inc.)

4. Banks, B. and Kenny, D. (1979). Looking at Sails. (Boston: Sail Books Inc.)

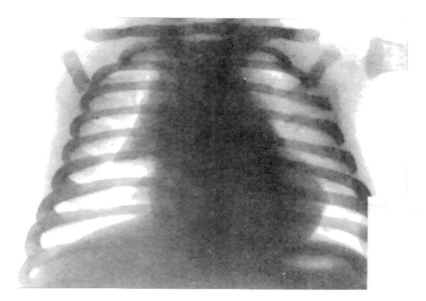

Figure 1. Chest radiograph with sail-like thymus. Reprinted from Kemp *et al.*[1] A sail-like triangular projection from the mediastinum a radiographic appearance of the thymus gland. *Br. J. Radiol.,* 1948, **21**, 618–624, with permission of the British Institute of Radiology

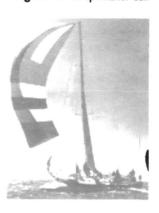

Figure 3. 'Crescentic sail-like shadow extending out over right lung and representing the displaced right lobe of the thymus.' Reprinted from Moseley[2]. Loculated pneumomediastinum in the newborn – a thymic 'spinnaker sail' sign. *Radiology,* 1960, **75**, 788–790, with permission of the RSNA

Figure 2. Sloop with triangular sails. Photo courtesy of United States Navy

Figure 4. A spinnaker sail

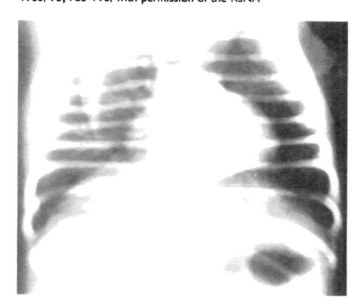

SAUSAGE (COCKTAIL SAUSAGE) DIGIT

Examination of the peripheral soft tissues often yields valuable clues to the radiologist who does not forget to inspect this part of the radiographic image. The appearance of a sausage digit (cocktail sausage digit) (Figure 1) is classically associated with the single-ray pattern of involvement seen in some patients with psoriatic arthritis. It may be the initial manifestation of the disease. This term is attributed, by Verna Wright and John Michael H. Moll[1], to Charles Bourdillon[2] who wrote his doctoral thesis on *Psoriasis et arthropathies* in 1888 with detailed accounts of 36 patients including descriptions of their swollen digits. Deborah Forrester, in a more recent article from UCLA-USC Medical Center, listed the differential diagnosis as trauma, cellulitis, osteomyelitis, the rheumatoid variant disorders and gout[3].

'Baron Jean Louis Alibert is often regarded as the first to mention the association between psoriasis and arthritis ... The name 'Psoriasis Arthritique' was coined by the celebrated skin physician Pierre Bazin in 1860.'[1] Although there is an association, a patient with psoriasis and arthritis does not necessarily have psoriatic arthritis. As a corollary, one may see the radiographic changes of psoriatic arthritis in a patient who does not have the dermatologic condition.

'Sausage is one of the oldest foods known to man [Figure 2]. Nobody knows who first thought of stuffing ground-up meat into a sheath, but Homer sang of sausage in the Odyssey, which was written (they say) about 850 BC. The Babylonians made and ate it, too ... Our word sausage stems from the Latin salsus, the word for salted or preserved meat.'[4]

References
1. Wright, V. and Moll, J.M.H. (1971). Psoriatic arthritis. *Bull. Rheum. Dis.*, 21, 627–32

2. Bourdillon, C. (1888). Psoriasis et arthropathies. (Paris: Lecrosnier et Babe)

3. Forrester, D.M. (1983). The 'cocktail sausage' digit. *Arthritis Rheum.*, 26, 664–7

4. Gehman, R. (1969). *The Sausage Book*, p. 6. (Englewood Cliffs, NJ: Prentice-Hall Inc.)

Figure 1. Radiograph showing diffuse soft tissue swelling around finger of patient with psoriatic arthritis. Case courtesy of Dr C. Resnik, University of Maryland

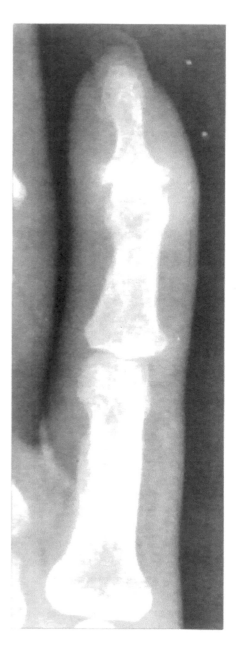

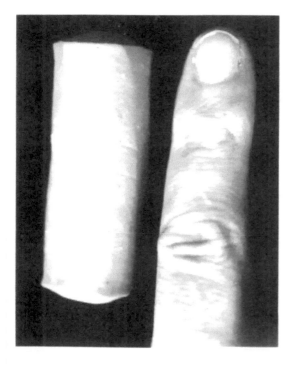

Figure 2. Cocktail sausage comparison with normal finger

SCIMITAR SIGN

The first detailed description of this pulmonary venous anomaly is said to be Edwards Albert Park's autopsy report[1] concerning a 2-month-old boy, published in 1912. This child was seen at the New York Foundling Hospital where he died about 2 weeks after admission. The scimitar term was not used in this report and there was no mention of an unusual vascular shadow in the description of the chest 'X-ray picture'. The vascular shadow was probably not evident on the X-ray due to severe hypoplasia of the right lung and shift of the heart into the right side of the chest. Park's clinical diagnosis was lobular pneumonia with the right lung 'consolidated in all but its upper part.' The autopsy showed a very small right pulmonary artery. No right pulmonary veins drained into the left auricle (atrium). Further examination revealed a large vein (the 'scimitar') receiving branches from both the right upper and lower lobes 'emptying into the inferior vena cava immediately at its point of emergence from the diaphragm.'[1]

John Roehm and colleagues[2] (University of Minnesota) describing the scimitar syndrome said, 'The full-blown syndrome, which invariably involves the right lung and its vascular supply, consists of: (a) hypoplasia of the right lung with subsequent dextroposition of the heart into the right thoracic cavity; (b) hypoplasia of the right pulmonary artery; (c) anomalous arterial supply from the abdominal aorta to the right lower lobe; (d) most important of all, anomalous venous drainage of the right lung by a large vein emptying into the inferior vena cava [Figure 1]. Due to its gentle curvature, the vein appears quite similar to a curved sword or scimitar.'

A scimitar is a short curved sword with a single edge, introduced in the sixteenth century, used especially by the Turks[3] (Figure 2). The word, scimitar, may be derived from the word, shamshir (shamsheer), according to The Royal Armouries, London.

References

1. Park, E.A. (1912). Defective development of the right lung, due to anomalous development of the right pulmonary artery and vein, accompanied by dislocation of the heart simulating dextrocardia. *Proc. New York Path. Soc.*, 12, 88–93

2. Roehm, J.O.F., Jue, K.L. and Amplatz, K. (1966). Radiographic features of the scimitar syndrome. *Radiology*, 86, 856–9

3. Burton, R.F (1884). *The Book of the Sword*, pp. 123–39. (London: Chatto and Windus)

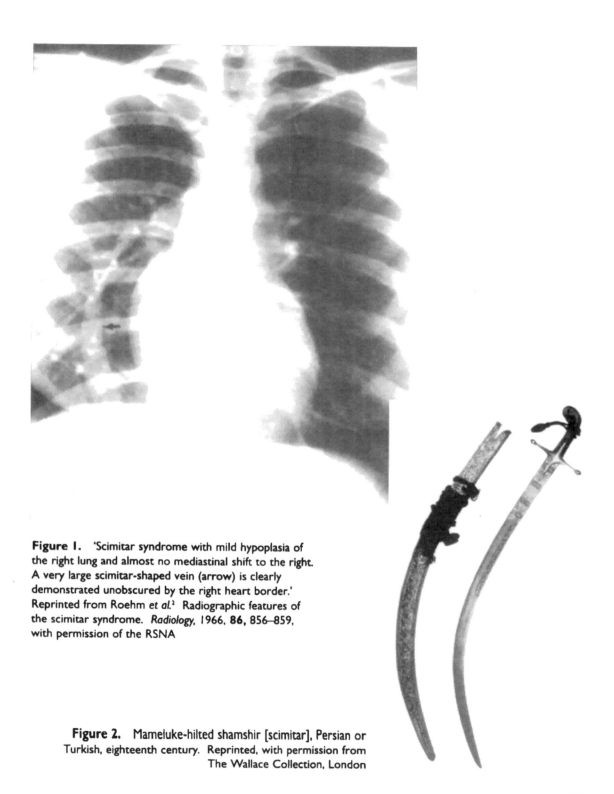

Figure 1. 'Scimitar syndrome with mild hypoplasia of the right lung and almost no mediastinal shift to the right. A very large scimitar-shaped vein (arrow) is clearly demonstrated unobscured by the right heart border.' Reprinted from Roehm *et al.*[2] Radiographic features of the scimitar syndrome. *Radiology,* 1966, **86,** 856–859, with permission of the RSNA

Figure 2. Mameluke-hilted shamshir [scimitar], Persian or Turkish, eighteenth century. Reprinted, with permission from The Wallace Collection, London

SCOTTIE DOG SIGN

'With a little imagination,' one can detect the form of a small dog in the outline of a lumbar vertebral body's parts as seen on an oblique radiograph (Figure 1). This simple observation, reported by A.-P. Lachapèle[1] in 1938, has provided radiologists with an easy method of remembering the complex anatomy in this crucial area. Lachapèle (Hôpital Saint-André de Bordeaux) compared the anatomic outline to Pol Rab's cartoon character Scottish terrier 'Rac'[2] (Figures 2 and 3), thus giving us the 'Scottie dog.' The most important feature is the 'neck' of the Scottie dog. This corresponds to the pars interarticularis and it is the site of abnormality when spondylolysis is present. A break in the neck of the dog or a collar on the dog's neck is indicative of spondylolysis. In the very next article in the journal Lachapèle[3] discussed cases of spondylolysis and illustrated how the 'Scottie dog' analogy applies to the radiographic findings. A renewed emphasis was placed on the importance of spondylolysis detection in the 1950s because of the increased use of preplacement lumbar spine X-rays for industrial workers and heavy laborers.

'The Scottish terrier [Figure 4], also called Scottie, is a short-legged terrier breed often held ... to be the oldest of the Highland terriers'[4]. 'What is probably the earliest reference to this little working terrier of Scotland refers to a 'wiry-haired Scotch terrier' in 1813.'[5]

References

1. Lachapèle, A.P. (1939). Un moyen simple pour faciliter la lecture des radiographies vertébrales obliques de la région lombo-sacrée. *Bull. Mem. Soc. Electro-radiol. Med. France*, 27, 175–6

2. Rab, P. (1930). *'Pas Pour Jeunes Filles': 125 Réflexions de Ric et Rac.* (Paris: Arthème Fayard and Cie)

3. Lachapèle, A.P. (1939). A propos de glissements vertebraux. *Bull. Mem. Soc. Electro-radiol. Med. France*, 27, 176–9

4. Scottish terrier. In *The New Encyclopaedia Britannica*, 1990, 15th edn, Vol. 10, p. 567. (Chicago: Encyclopaedia Britannica Inc.)

5. Caspersz, D.S. (1976). *The Scottish Terrier*, p.7. (New York: Arco Publishing Co. Inc.)

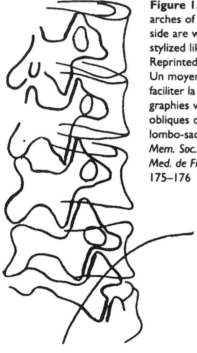

Figure 1. 'The posterior arches of the examined side are whimsically stylized like a small dog.' Reprinted from Lachapèle[1]. Un moyen simple pour faciliter la lecture des radiographies vertébrales obliques de la région lombo-sacrée. Bull et Mem. Soc. Electro-radiol. Med. de France, 1939, **27**, 175–176

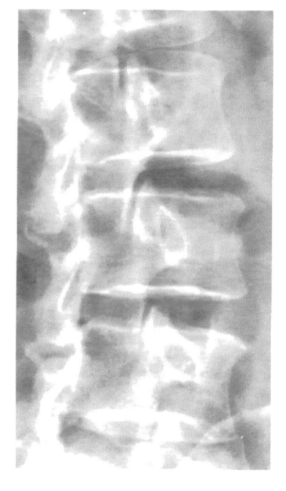

Figure 2. Posterior oblique radiograph of lumbar spine showing the Scottie dog (author's case)

Figure 3. Pol Rab's dog 'Rac'. Reprinted from 'Pas Pour Jeunes Filles': 125 Réflexions de Ric et Rac by Rab (1930)[2], published by Arthème Fayard and Cie, Paris

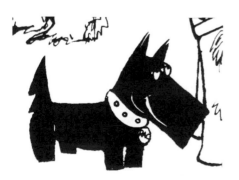

Figure 4. Champion Scottish Terrier Carmichael's Fanfare. Reproduced courtesy of E. Kirks of The Scottish Terrier Club of America, Roanoke, VA

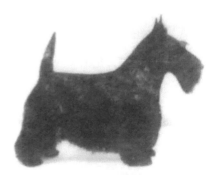

SHEPHERD'S CROOK

This deformity of the proximal femur, classically associated with fibrous dysplasia, was described by Friedrich von Recklinghausen[1] (1833–1910) in 1891. His patient was a 66-year-old woman who came to medical attention because of a pneumonia. On physical examination she was noted to have a 'shepherd's crook curvature [hirtenstabförmige] of both femurs.' The cause of the femoral deformity in this woman was not explained. The ray that would shed light on many of the unknowns for physicians, the X-ray, was discovered 4 years later.

The shepherd's crook femur is now recognized as a consequence of any condition that causes deformity, softening or fragility of the bones. In addition to fibrous dysplasia, some of the more common conditions that may lead to a shepherd's crook deformity include Paget's disease, osteogenesis imperfecta and renal osteodystrophy or other osteomalacic disorders (Figure 1).

Osteomalacia also greatly interested von Recklinghausen. In the same group of clinical cases that included the shepherd's-crook discussion he gave the first detailed description of patients with what he called *osteitis fibrosa cystica*. This is the old descriptive pathology name for the disorder that we now know is due to hyperparathyroidism.

One definition of a crook is, 'A shepherd's staff, having one end curved or hooked, for catching the hinder [hind] leg of a sheep'[2] (Figure 2).

References

1. von Recklinghausen, F. (1891). Die Fibröse oder deformierende Ostitis, die Osteomalacie und die osteoplastische Carcinose in ihren gegenseitigen Beziehungen. In *Festschrift; Rudolf Virchow zu seinem 71.* (Berlin: Reimer–Berlin)

2. Crook. In Simpson, J. and Weiner, E. *Oxford English Dictionary*, 1989, 2nd edn, Vol. 4, p. 39. (Oxford: Clarendon Press)

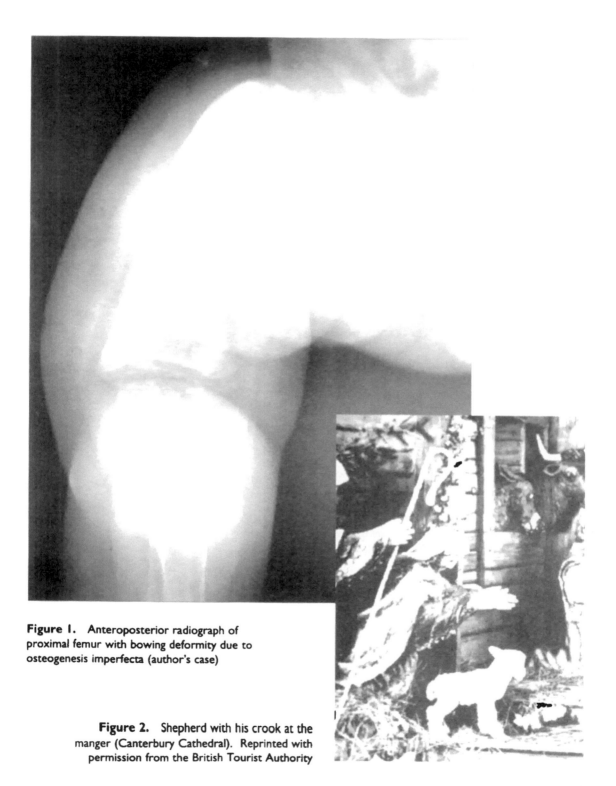

Figure 1. Anteroposterior radiograph of proximal femur with bowing deformity due to osteogenesis imperfecta (author's case)

Figure 2. Shepherd with his crook at the manger (Canterbury Cathedral). Reprinted with permission from the British Tourist Authority

SHMOO SHAPED HEART

Making the correct diagnosis in cases of congenital heart disease has always been challenging. This is especially true at the viewbox when one has only a chest radiograph and some limited clinical information (cyanotic or not cyanotic) to go on. Careful analysis of many factors including assessment of the pulmonary vascularity (increased, normal or decreased), size and position of the aorta, aortic knob, pulmonary artery and left ventricle is essential. Larry Elliott[1] (University of Florida in 1968), credited a former teacher, Lewis Carey (University of Minnesota), for the analogy of an enlarged left ventricle to one of Al Capp's 'Shmoos'. 'The left ventricular configuration is remembered more easily by the beginning student if it is considered or likened to Al Capp's 'Shmoo.'[1] When left ventricular enlargement is combined with an ectatic ascending aorta, especially in the setting of aortic insufficiency, the Shmoo-shaped heart is most evident (Figures 1 and 2), in this author's opinion. Cardiac shapes with either ventricular hypertrophy or ventricular enlargement were originally associated with the variable shape of a shmoo and are illustrated in the book[1].

The Shmoo was a comic strip creature that was featured in Al Capp's 'Li'l Abner.' It was described as: 'a small white squash with two tiny legs, a pair of eyes and wispy mustache hairs. Nothing else. It was a rather amorphous object.'[2]

References
1. Elliott, L.P. and Schiebler, G.L. (1968). *X-ray Diagnosis of Congenital Cardiac Disease*, p. 109. (Springfield: Charles C. Thomas)

2. Capp, A. (1959). *The Return of the Shmoo*. (New York: Simon & Schuster)

3. Capp, A. (1949). *The Life and Times of the Shmoo*. (New York: Pocket Books)

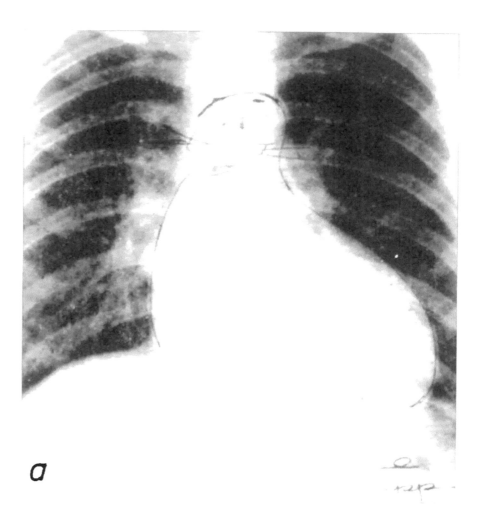

a

Figure 1. 'Drawing of 'Shmoo' on PA film in patient with left ventricular enlargement. This was done through the courtesy of Al Capp to dramatize the likeness of left ventricular disease to the configuration of the Shmoo.' Reprinted from *X-ray Diagnosis of Congenital Cardiac Disease* by Elliott and Schiebler (1968)[1], with permission of Charles C Thomas, Publisher, Springfield,Il

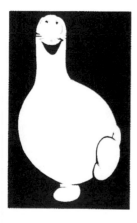

Figure 2. One of Al Capp's Shmoos. Reprinted with permission from *The Life and Times of the Shmoo* by Capp (1949)[3], published by Pocket Books, New York. © Capp Enterprises Inc. All rights reserved

SHOTGUN (PARALLEL CHANNEL) SIGN

In 1978, two ultrasonographic signs of biliary-tree obstruction were published. One was called the 'parallel channel' sign by Melvyn Conrad and colleagues[1] (Parkland Memorial Hospital, Dallas), since the simultaneous appearance of dilated right or left main hepatic ducts and the accompanying portal vein branches resulted in an ultrasound image with parallel channels. The second was named the 'shotgun' sign by Francis Weill and co-workers[2], presumably with a double-barrel shotgun in mind, since it also described the visualization of side-by-side tubular structures. In this case, the main bile duct (denoting common hepatic and common bile duct) and the portal vein were the side-by-side structures (Figure 1). When the main bile duct was seen to be equal to or greater in size than the portal vein, this was deemed an early sign of biliary-tree obstruction. 'Since it is now possible to visualize at least the proximal segment of the biliary tree with regularity, the diagnosis of early dilatation of the biliary tree is possible. Normally, the biliary junction is narrower than the portal vein or the portal division. With early dilatation the two diameters tend to equalize. Thus, the presence of two parallel channels with similar diameters (which we call the 'shotgun' sign) is pathologic.'[2] It was found to be a valuable criterion for differentiating obstructive from non-obstructive jaundice in a study of 100 cases[2].

It is fitting that the shotgun sign was described by these three European physicians (University Hospital [CHU], Besançon, France) because the earliest smooth-bore firearms loaded with shot (shotguns) were the fowling pieces that appeared in sixteenth century Europe[3]. Double-barrel shotguns come in either side-by-side or over-and-under styles (Figure 2).

References
1. Conrad, M.R., Landay, M.J. and Janes, J.O. (1978). Sonographic 'parallel channel' sign of biliary tree enlargement in mild to moderate obstructive jaundice. *Am. J. Roentgenol.*, 130, 279–86

2. Weill, F., Eisencher, A. and Zeltner, F. (1978). Ultrasonic study of the normal and dilated biliary tree. *Radiology*, 127, 221–4

3. Shotgun. In *The New Encyclopaedia Britannica*, 15th edn, Vol. 10, p. 764. (Chicago: Encyclopaedia Britannica Inc.)

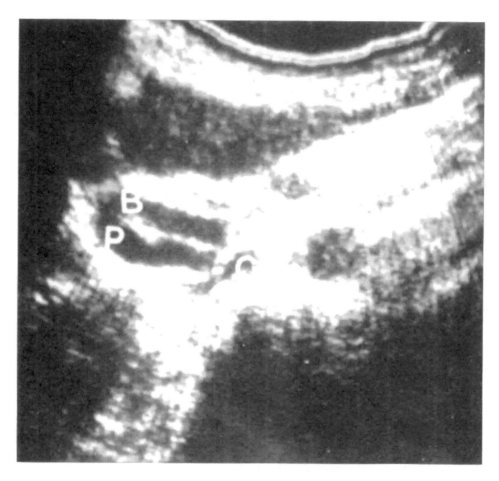

Figure 1. 'This transverse scan of the liver with the transducer angled cephalad shows the biliary junction and a proximal segment of the main bile duct (B) in front of the hilar division of the portal vein (P). The diameter of the bile duct is equal to that of the portal vein. (C = vena cava).' Reprinted from Weill et al.[2] Ultrasonic study of the normal and dilated biliary tree. *Radiology* 1978, **127**, 221–224, with permission of the RSNA

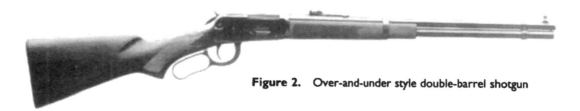

Figure 2. Over-and-under style double-barrel shotgun

SILHOUETTE SIGN

There are classics and then there are *classics*. In addition to classic signs, there are classic radiologists. Benjamin (Ben) Felson (1913–1988) was one of the most outstanding radiologists and teachers of our times. The silhouette sign that he and his brother Henry[1] reported in 1950, will forever be associated with the Felson name though they stated that several others had discussed the phenomenon before their report[2-4].

The Felsons (University of Cincinnati, Ohio) stated, 'With the rapid advances in thoracic surgery, segmental localization of pulmonary disease has assumed greater importance'. [Their method of determining] 'the exact location of a pulmonary density from the postero–anterior film alone' [was] 'based on the premise that an intra-thoracic radiopacity, if in *anatomic* contact with a border of the heart or aorta, [would] obscure that border.' [They] 'adopted the term *silhouette sign* to indicate obliteration of a portion of the cardiovascular silhouette by adjacent disease' (Figure 1). They tested this premise experimentally and with a study of 84 patients. The sign proved to be very reliable and has withstood the test of time. There has been a lot of discussion about whether this sign should be called a 'silhouette sign' or a 'loss of the silhouette sign.' The term, silhouette sign, ought to be remembered as it was defined by its originators with fewer arguments about the semantics involved.

'The word 'silhouette' originated in France and denotes shadows seen against light – or, in modern usage, outlined forms [Figure 2]; it is derived from the name of Etienne de Silhouette (1709–1769), a frugal and heartily disliked minister of finance under Louis XV, whose favourite hobby was the cutting of profiles from black paper. Some years after his death, de Silhouette's name was applied derisively to the pastime he had enjoyed.'[5,6]

References

1. Felson, B. and Felson, H. (1950). Localization of intra-thoracic lesions by means of the postero–anterior roentgenogram. *Radiology,* 55, 363–74

2. Dunham, H.K. Cited by Felson, B. and Felson, H.[1] (1950), as a personal communication

3. Robbins, L.L. and Hale, C.H. (1945). The roentgen appearance of lobar and segmental collapse of the lung. *Radiology,* 44, 107–14 and 45, 120–7, 260–6, 347–55

4. Hampton, A.O. and King, D.S. (1936). The middle lobe of the right lung. Its roentgen appearance in health and disease. *Am. J. Roentgenol.*, 35, 721–39

5. Hickman, P. (1975). *Silhouettes – A Living Art*, p. 10. (London: David and Charles Ltd)

6. Carrick, van leer, A. (1928). *Shades of our Ancestors.* (Boston: Little, Brown & Co.)

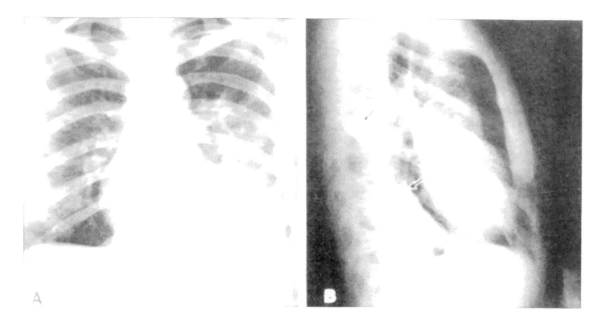

Figure 1. Silhouette sign seen in 'tuberculosis with cavitation, bronchostenosis, and collapse. A. In the postero-anterior view the preservation of the left heart border indicates lower lobe disease. B. Left lateral view confirms the localization (arrows).' Reprinted from Felson and Felson[1]. Localization of intrathoracic lesions by means of PA roentgenogram. *Radiology*, 1950, **55**, 363–374, with permission of the RSNA

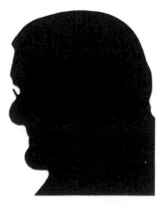

Figure 2. Ben Felson in silhouette on X-ray film

SILVER FORK DEFORMITY

The most common fracture of the distal radius in the adult is Colles' fracture (Figure 1). Although Abraham Colles[1] (1773–1843) thought his 1814 report was the first to describe this injury, it had in fact been described earlier by Claude Pouteau[2] (1725–1775), chief surgeon of the Hôtel Dieu in Lyon. 'In a memoir published posthumously in 1783 ... [Pouteau] described the fracture of the distal end of the radius with posterior tipping or displacement of the distal fragment.'[3] Neither of these authors used the term silver-fork deformity in their descriptions of this injury, although Colles (Steeven's Hospital, Dublin) did accurately describe it as 'The posterior surface of the limb presents a considerable deformity; for a depression is seen in the forearm, about an inch and a half above the end of this bone, [radius] while a considerable swelling occupies the wrist and the metacarpus. Indeed the carpus and base of metacarpus appear to be thrown backward so much, as on first view to excite a suspicion that the carpus has been dislocated forward.'[1] It was 'Alfred Armand Velpeau (1795–1867) [who] termed the usual deformity seen in fractures of the distal end of the radius the talon de fourchette which, translated into English, meant the 'silver fork deformity'.'[3]

The work of these surgeons (Pouteau, Colles, Velpeau) was instrumental in correcting the misconception that existed 'from the time of Hippocrates to the beginning of the nineteenth century, [namely that] fractures of the distal end of the radius were ... dislocations of the wrist.'[3]

'The fork is the most recent addition to the family of table implements ... and was first used as a table implement in Italy ... as early as about the year 1000 ... But it was not until the end of the

seventeenth century that the final form commonly known as the 'French fork' [Figure 2] – curved and with three (or more often four) short prongs – made its appearance.'[4]

References

1. Colles, A. (1814). On the fracture of the carpal extremity of the radius. *Edinburgh Med. Surg. J.*, 10, 182–6

2. Pouteau, C. (1783). Contenant quelques réflexions sur quelques fractures de l'avant-bras sur le luxations incomplettes du poignet et sur le diastasis. In *Oeuveres Posthumes de M. Pouteau*, Book 2, pp. 251–66. (Paris: Ph.-D. Pierres)

3. Peltier, L.F. (1984). Fractures of the distal end of the radius: an historical account. *Clin. Orthop.*, 187, 18–22

4. Brunner, H. (1967). *Old Table Silver*, 1st edn, p. 59. (New York: Taplinger Publishing Co. Inc.)

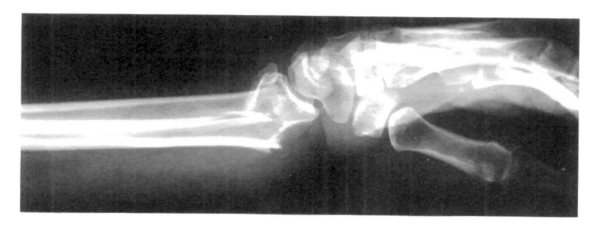

Figure 1. Lateral radiograph showing typical Colles' fracture with silver-fork deformity (author's case)

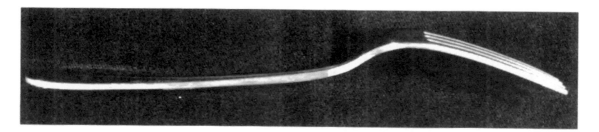

Figure 2. A silver dinner fork. Courtesy of Mr E.L. Mulligan

SNOWMAN (FIGURE-8) SIGN

An 'increasing interest in abnormal venous return' seems to have prompted H.A. Snellen and F.H. Albers[1] (University Hospital, Leiden) to report their experience with five cases in 1952. Four of their five cases had 'total abnormal pulmonary venous drainage (via 'left vena cava' and left innominate vein into the superior vena cava on the right side)' with a characteristic roentgenographic configuration that they termed the figure-8 (Figure 1). In the discussion of their second case they said, 'On both sides of the upper mediastinum a large rounded shadow was seen to bulge into the lung fields; the right shadow was more prominent than the left ... With the heart shadow they formed a figure-8 shaped mass.'[1] Their diagnoses were confirmed with angiocardiography that showed the top of the figure-8 to be composed of the draining veins with the bottom portion formed by the heart. They noted that many earlier articles had discussed similar cases but emphasized that the conventional chest roentgenogram could make the diagnosis with near complete certainty. The figure-8 sign is often referred to now as the snowman sign (Figure 2).

Our numerals (1–9) are Hindu-Arabic in origin. They can be traced to 'the Brâhmî system of numeral writing, established by decree of the Emperor Aśoka (c. 250 BC), [where] each unit receives one individual symbol, one figure.' They became known to the West by way of Spain. 'Spain was, with Sicily, the only European country which had been under the Arabs for centuries. The oldest extant European manuscript with the new figures comes from the Albedo monastery ... in northern Spain, and dates from AD 976.'[2]

References

1. Snellen, H.A. and Albers, F.H. (1952). The clinical diagnosis of anomalous pulmonary venous drainage. *Circulation*, 6, 801–16

2. Flegg, G. (ed.) (1989). *Numbers Through the Ages*, pp. 105–16. (London: Macmillan Education Ltd)

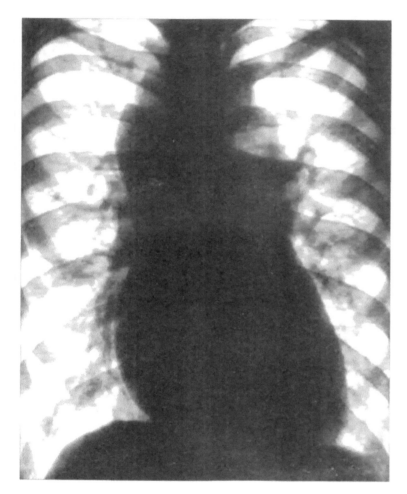

Figure 1. Anteroposterior view of chest with 'saccular bulging of both sides of the upper mediastinum.' Reprinted from Snellen and Albers'. The clinical diagnosis of anomalous pulmonary venous drainage. *Circulation*, 1952, **6**, 801–816, with permission of the American Heart Association

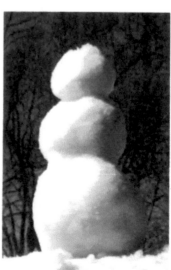

Figure 2. A snowman

SPINNING TOP (ARROWHEAD) URETHRA

Exhaustive investigations of the bladder and urethra have been performed to explain the cause of urinary tract infection in young girls. Richards Lyon (UCSF) and his colleagues[1,2] did some of the most in depth work and reported their findings, from a large group of girls, in articles that appeared in the *Journal of Urology* in 1963 and 1965. The initial study group of 100 girls discussed in the 1963 article had grown to 152 at the time of the 1965 report. Voiding cystourethrograms for these patients showed many different proximal urethral shapes which included: funnel, arrowhead (spinning top) and T-shape (Figure 1). These shapes were all thought to be indicative of urethral stenosis. The spinning top urethra and its alternate forms became very controversial signs since many other authors felt that they were normal findings. This latter opinion has prevailed and the appearance of a spinning top urethra is now considered normal.

A top is 'a toy having a body of conical, circular, or oval shape, often hollow, with a point or peg on which it turns or is made to whirl [Figure 2]. Tops were known to the ancient Greeks and Romans ... The top was known in Europe as early as the 14th century.'[3]

References

1. Lyon, R.P and Smith, D.R. (1963). Distal urethral stenosis. *J. Urol.*, **89**, 414–21

2. Lyon, R.P and Tanagho, E.A. (1965). Distal urethral stenosis in little girls. *J. Urol.*, **93**, 379–87

3. Top. In *The New Encyclopaedia Britannica*, 1990, 15th edn, Vol. 11, p. 847. (Chicago: Encyclopaedia Britannica Inc.)

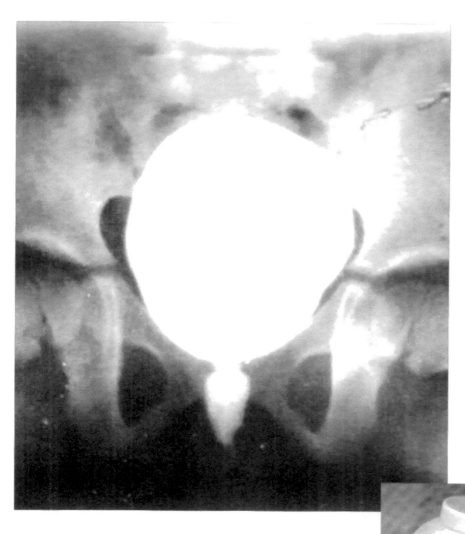

Figure 1. Arrowhead (spinning top) outline in child with 'distal urethral stenosis.' Reprinted from Lyon and Tanagho[2]. Distal urethral stenosis in little girls. *J. Urol.,* 1965, **93**, 379–87, with permission of Williams and Wilkins

Figure 2. A toy top

STAGHORN CALCULI

Hippocrates (460–375 BC) specifically mentions pain starting in the kidney or kidney region and radiating to the testicle and to the presence of kidney stones. Riolan, in the first half of the seventeenth century is, according to Legueu, the first writer to speak of renal calculi in a precise manner. He recognized their coral-like form and was aware of their position in the ureter, the pelvis and the calices[1]. Large coral-like stones were also called branched or staghorn calculi[2] (Figure 1).

The first report of a renal stone seen by roentgen photography was from Glasgow by John MacIntyre[3] in July 1896. This was only 6 months after the news of Roentgen's discovery had been announced in England. Much of the early experience with the new X-rays involved pictures of the extremities, since they were easy to immobilize for the requisite long-exposure times. MacIntyre's feat of obtaining good quality pictures of the abdomen is enviable even today. He described the roentgen photographic technique he used to visualize a renal stone in a patient referred to him by James Adams from the Glasgow Royal Infirmary. Adams confirmed the radiographic finding after a successful operation to remove the stone. (Some authors have mistakenly credited Adams with the roentgenographic 'first'.)

Most stags' 'horns' are not horns at all, they are antlers. Horns 'consist of a non-deciduous cuticle composed of keratin. Antlers are outgrowths of bone. [Antlers] are carried by most members of the deer family and, with the exception of reindeer and caribou, are limited to the stags only'[4] (Figure 2).

References
1. Barney, J.D. (1933). Lithiasis. In Lewis, B. (ed.) *History of Urology*, pp. 15–16. (Baltimore: Williams & Wilkins Company)

2. Young, H.H. and Waters, C.A. (1928). Urinary lithiasis. In *Urological Roentgenology*, pp. 302–413. (New York: Paul Hoeber)

3. MacIntyre, J. (1896). Photography of renal calculus. *Lancet*, ii, 118

4. MacGregor, A. (1985). *Bone, Antler, Ivory and Horn*, pp. 9–20. (London: Croom Helm Ltd)

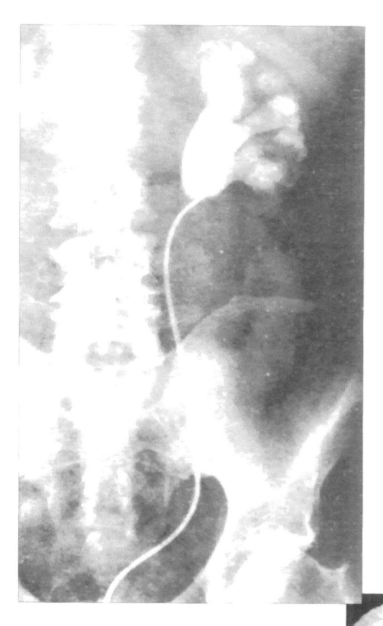

Figure 1. 'Huge stag-horn calculus, completely filling pelvis and calices.' Reprinted from Young and Waters (1928)[2]. Urinary lithiasis. In *Urological Roentgenology*, published by Paul Hoeber, New York

Figure 2. Alaskan moose antler

STRING SIGN

Only 2 years after Burrill Crohn and colleagues[1] described regional ileitis as a pathologic and clinical entity (see Cobblestone pattern), John Kantor[2] reported its diagnostic roentgenographic features. Kantor worked with the same surgeons and pathologists as Crohn and his colleagues[1]. His report was based on six cases and included a description of the 'string sign' (Figure 1). 'Perhaps the most striking finding is the 'string sign' ... This is a thin, slightly irregular linear shadow suggesting a cotton string in appearance and extending more or less continuously from the region of the last visualized loop of ileum through the entire extent of the filling defect and ending at the ileocecal valve. It represents the attenuated barium filling of the greatly contracted intestinal lumen. A characteristic 'string sign' is apparent in the illustration of the original article by Crohn and his collaborators.'[2] Kantor said the name 'string sign' was 'borrowed from A.W. Crane.' In the discussion that followed Kantor's article, Crohn endorses the sign saying, 'It is a fitting term. The string sign is absolutely characteristic.' Kantor, however, did not consider it to be a pathognomonic sign. Tuberculomas, syphilitic colitis and stenosing sarcomas of the terminal ileum had also been reported with a similar radiographic appearance.

String is a 'line for binding or attaching anything, normally one composed of twisted threads of spun vegetable fibre'[3] (Figure 2).

References

1. Crohn, B.B., Ginzburg, L. and Oppenheimer, G.D. (1932). Regional ileitis – a pathologic and clinical entity. *J. Am. Med. Assoc.*, 99, 1323–9

2. Kantor, J.L. (1934). Regional (terminal) ileitis: its roentgen diagnosis. *J. Am. Med. Assoc.*, 103, 2016–21

3. String. In Simpson, J. and Weiner, E. (eds.) *Oxford English Dictionary*, 2nd edn., Vol. 16, p. 920. (Oxford: Clarendon Press)

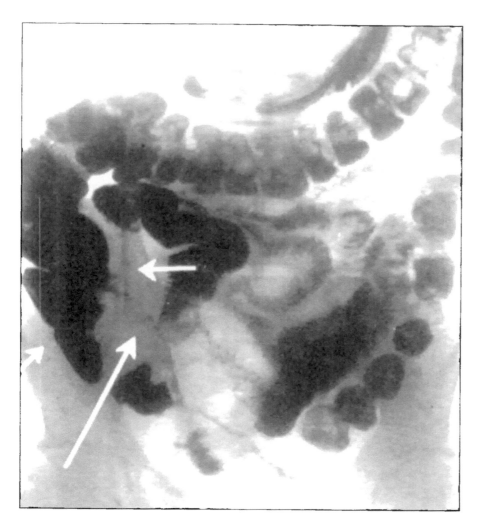

Figure 1. 'Regional (terminal) ileitis, showing multiple
string signs.' Reprinted from Kantor². Regional (terminal)
ileitis. *J. Am. Med. Assoc.*, 1934, **103**, 2016–2021, copyright
1934, American Medical Association

Figure 2. Household string

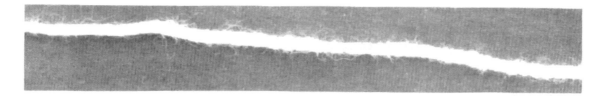

SUNBURST PATTERN

One of the earliest and most eloquent descriptions of the characteristic periosteal reaction seen with osteosarcomas was that of Frederick Baetjer[1] (Johns Hopkins University). In the 1921 textbook, he wrote with Charles Waters, he referred to the radiating spicules of periosteal sarcoma as 'resembling the rays of the sunset' and those of central osteosarcoma 'like church spires piercing a city's sky line'[1] (Figure 1). For osteosarcomas, this sunray pattern has been transformed, in today's terminology, into a sunburst. This is perhaps more in keeping with the aggressive (malignant) growth indicated by this sign. The sunray terminology is still used, more appropriately in this author's opinion, for the appearance of a benign lesion, a hemangioma in the skull. Many other authors used the radiating spicule and ray terminology before Baetjer and certainly influenced him[2].

Baetjer (1874–1933) was one of the first radiologists to teach a systematic approach for the diagnosis of bone tumors. The development of his organized approach was no doubt prompted by his duties as an X-ray instructor for the United States Army during World War I. Baetjer ran a school at Cornell University where 'several hundred physicians were prepared for X-ray work in the United States Army in a little over 1 year.'[3] Baetjer's analysis of bone tumors included a determination of: origin, medullary or cortical; bone production or destruction; the condition of the cortex, expanded or destroyed; and an assessment of the invasiveness of the tumor. This approach was also undoubtedly influenced by his association, before the war, with surgical colleagues at Johns Hopkins University, especially Joseph Bloodgood (1867–1935).

Our sun is estimated to be about 5 billion years old. It's rays do burst forth at times (Figure 2). The largest bursts or flames 'protruding into dark space ... are called prominences. Our own star is only one of perhaps 100 billion stars which shine in the [Milky Way] Galaxy today. Astronomers estimate that there are at least 100 billion galaxies, similar in stellar content to our own, in the known universe.'[4]

References
1. Baetjer, F.H. and Waters, C.A. (1921). Bone tumors. In *Injuries and Diseases of the Bones and Joints*, pp. 263–6. (New York: Paul B. Hoeber Inc.)

2. Bloodgood, J.C. (1903). Benign and malignant tumors of bone. *Prog. Med.*, 4, 186–204

3. Nichols, B.H. (1922). Roentgen diagnosis of the more important tumors of the long bones. *Surg. Gynecol. Obstet.*, 35, 301–9

4. Noyes, R.W. (1982). *The Sun, Our Star*, pp. 1–120. (Cambridge, MA: Harvard University Press)

5. Lodwick, G.S. (1971). *The Bones and Joints*. (Chicago: Year Book Medical Publishers)

Figure 1. Osteosarcoma with 'Lumps, clouds and consolidated rays of tumor bone in the upper half of the extraosseous mass.' Reprinted with permission from *The Bones and Joints* by Lodwick (1971)[5], published by Year Book Medical Publishers, Chicago. Copyright 1971 by the ACR

Figure 2. 'A relatively small prominence [sunburst] extending about 50 000 kilometers (4 Earth diameters) above the solar limb.' Courtesy of the National Solar Observatory/Sacramento Peak, NM

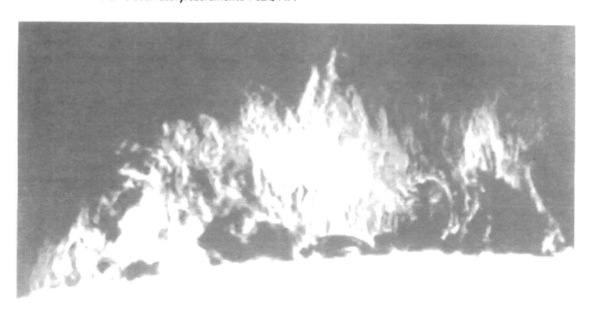

TEAR-DROP (PEAR-SHAPED) BLADDER

Trauma is not responsible for many of the radiologic signs in this book. However, one of the classics is the traumatically induced tear-drop or pear-shaped bladder. George Prather and Thomas Kaiser[1] (Boston City Hospital) used the term tear-drop bladder in their 1950 article describing '[t]wo recent cases of pelvic fracture, showing in the opaque cystogram a narrow and elongated configuration which we have dubbed 'tear-drop bladder'. We believe [this] is caused by extensive perivesical hemorrhage'[1] (Figure 1). Extensive pelvic hematoma was indeed found to be the cause of the abnormal bladder configuration. Marjorie Ambos and her colleagues[2] (New York University) used the term 'pear-shaped' and expanded the etiologic list in their 1977 article. Pelvic lipomatosis, inferior vena cava occlusion, lymphocysts and pelvic lymphadenopathy were other causes for the abnormal bladder shape that they discussed. In addition, they described other findings that might allow a specific diagnosis to be made.

'The most important genera of pome fruits (Family Rosaceae, Subfamily Pomoideae, x=17) are *Malus* (apple), *Pyrus* (pear), and *Cydonia* (quince) ... The genus *Pyrus* consists of about twenty species ... The domestic pear of Europe [Figure 2], like the apple, has been selected, improved and cultured since prehistoric times ... Written records exist from 1100 BC describing selection and culture of ... pears.'[3]

'No fruit has so many forms as the pear in its different varieties ... pyriform, obovate, and oblate, ... constitute the three principal divisions.'[4] Certainly, the bladder distorted by hematoma after trauma may take on nearly any of the pear's different forms.

References

1. Prather, G.C. and Kaiser, T.F. (1950). The bladder in fracture of the bony pelvis; the significance of a 'tear drop bladder' as shown by cystogram. *J. Urol.*, 63, 1019–30

2. Ambos, M.A., Bosniak, M.A., Lefleur, R.S. and Madayag, M.A. (1977). The pear-shaped bladder. *Radiology*, 122, 85–8

3. Westwood, M.N. (1978). *Temperate-zone Pomology*, pp. 41–5. (San Francisco: W.H. Freeman and Company)

4. Thomas, J.J. (1897). *The American Fruit Culturist*, 20th edn, p. 442. (New York: William Wood and Company)

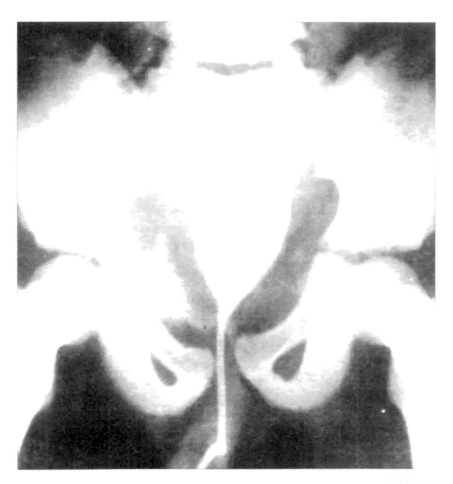

Figure 1. 'Cystogram obtained during intra-venous urography and retrograde injection. Bladder shows 'tear-drop' shape which is primarily caused by perivesical blood and urine.' Reprinted from Prather and Kaiser[1]. The bladder in fracture of the bony pelvis; the significance of a 'tear drop bladder' as shown by cystogram. *J. Urol.,* **63,** 1019–30, with permission of Williams & Wilkins

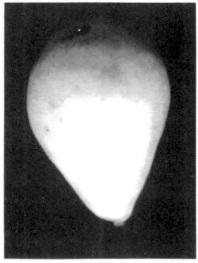

Figure 2. An Anjou pear

TELEPHONE RECEIVER FEMUR

Thantophoric dwarfism (thanatophoric dysplasia) was described in 1967 by Pierre Maroteaux and colleagues[1] (Hôpital des Enfants-Malades, Paris). They reported their findings in four cases and discussed the differential diagnostic features especially with regard to achondroplasia. One of the features they emphasized in this new disorder was the extreme shortening of the long bones. They also described the abnormal curvature of the diaphysis and the cupping, or flaring, and irregularity of the metaphysis (Figure 1). Four years later these abnormal features of the femurs were characterized as resembling a telephone receiver (Figure 2) by Joseph A. Bailey II (Johns Hopkins University) in his 1971 review article entitled, *Forms of Dwarfism Recognizable at Birth*. Bailey said, 'Affected individuals can be diagnosed even *in utero* on the basis of their characteristic bony deformities. Femurs shaped like 'telephone receivers' are an obvious feature.'[2] Simply put by Bailey, 'that's the way it appeared to me' (personal communication).

Alexander Graham Bell (1847–1922) invented the telephone in 1875[3]. Bell telephone receivers from the 1940s–1950s were similar in appearance to the long bones of a thanatophoric (death bringing) dwarf (Figure 2).

Thanatos was, in Greek mythology, the embodiment of Death himself. Thus, Thanatos is known as the Greek god of death. Applying his name to the peculiar form of dysplasia described above is appropriate, since most of these infants die within a very short period of time if they are not stillborn.

References

1. Maroteaux, P., Lamy, M. and Robert, J.M. (1967). Le Nanisme Thanatophore. *Presse Med.*, 75, 2519–24

2. Bailey, J.A. (1971). Forms of dwarfism recognizable at birth. *Clin. Orthop.*, 76, 150–9

3. Watson, T.A. (1977). How Bell invented the telephone. In Shiers G. (ed.) *The Telephone – An Historical Anthology*, pp. 1503–8. (New York: Arno Press)

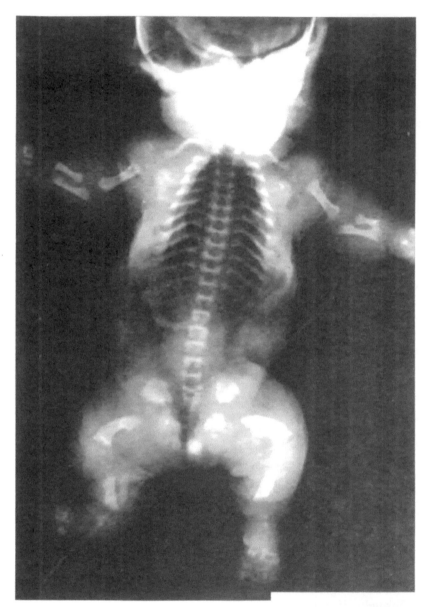

Figure 1.
'Thanatophoric Dwarfs:
The femora are shaped
like 'telephone-receivers'
because of the curved
diaphysis.' Reprinted from
Bailey[2]. Forms of
dwarfism recognizable at
birth. *Clin. Orthop.*, 1971,
76, 150–159, with
permission of J.B.
Lippincott Co.

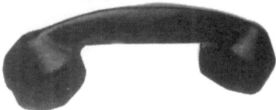

Figure 2. Receiver from 1940's
era Bell telephone

TERRY-THOMAS AND SIGNET RING SIGNS

'The application of anthropomorphic similies supplies us with diagnostic clues and triggers that simplify the complicated and clarify the opaque' – easy for Victor Frankel[1] (then, University of Washington) to say, in his 1977 letter, explaining the Terry-Thomas sign.

Widening of the joint space between the scaphoid and lunate, seen with rotatory subluxation of the scaphoid (scapholunate dislocation) (Figure 1), was reminiscent of the gap between the British comedian Terry Thomas's teeth. One may wish to substitute the identical dental display of their own favorite famous or infamous celebrity (e.g. Lauren Hutton or Mike Tyson) for that of Terry-Thomas. Scapholunate dislocation is one of the injuries that may result from a fall on the outstretched hand (FOOSH). It is important to make the diagnosis because, when left untreated, it is a cause of chronic wrist pain and disability.

'Terry-Thomas, born Thomas Terry Hoar-Stevens on Bastille Day, 1911, in London, is well known to the aficionados of British comedy. He is a comedian who despite an upper central dental diastema has a winning and unforgettable smile. He also has a not-to-be-forgotten grimace [Figure 2].'[1]

Another important sign of scapholunate dislocation is the cortical-ring (or signet-ring) sign described by J. Jay Crittenden and colleagues[2] (United States Naval Hospital, Yokosuka, Japan), in 1970. They reported a case of bilateral rotational dislocation of the carpal naviculars in a 21-year-old Marine. The abnormal orientation of the scaphoid causes a superimposition of cortical shadows from the wrist and distal pole that simulates a signet ring (Figures 3 and 4).

Signet rings became dominant in Hellenistic and Roman times as a method for authenticating documents. They replaced the older cylinder seal and Egyptian scarab[3].

References
1. Frankel, V.H. (1977). The Terry-Thomas sign. *Clin. Orthop.*, 129, 321–2

2. Crittenden, J.J., Jones, D.M. and Santarelli, A.G. (1970). Bilateral rotational dislocation of the carpal navicular. *Radiology*, 94, 629–30

3. Sigillography. In *The New Encyclopaedia Britannica*, 1990, 15th edn, Vol. 20, pp. 611–14. (Chicago: Encyclopaedia Britannica Inc.)

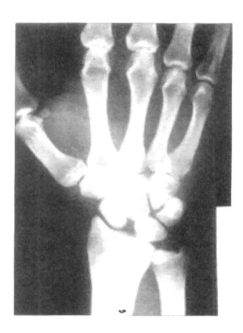

Figure 1. 'An antero-posterior radiograph showing rotational subluxation of the navicular, with a gap between the navicular and lunate.' Reprinted from Frankel[1]. The Terry-Thomas sign. *Clin. Orthop.*, 1977, **129**, 321–322, with permission of J.B. Lippincott Co.

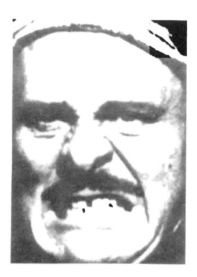

Figure 2. 'Dental diastema: facies (courtesy of Mr Terry-Thomas).' Reprinted from Frankel[1]. The Terry-Thomas sign. *Clin. Orthop.*, **129**, 321–2 with permission of Dr V.H. Frankel

Figure 3. Posteroanterior view shows 'rotational dislocation of the navicular' Reprinted from Crittenden et al.[2] Bilateral rotational dislocation of the carpal navicular. *Radiology*, 1970 **94**, 629–630, with permission of the RSNA

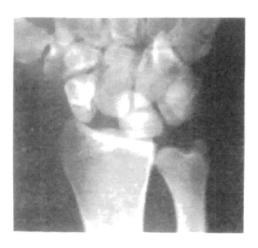

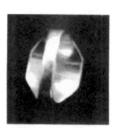

Figure 4. A signet ring

THUMBPRINTING SIGN

Thumbprinting as a sign of submucosal hemorrhage or edema in colonic vascular occlusion was reported in two articles by Scott Boley and colleagues[1] and Solomon Schwartz and co-workers[2], in 1963. The first article described the barium enema findings in five patients seen at the Jewish Hospital of Brooklyn and Downstate Medical Center (Figure 1). 'The roentgenologic finding of importance is pseudotumor formation or 'thumbprinting'. This appears to be caused by submucosal hemorrhage or by pericolic fat inflammation or both.'[1] The second article detailed the course of the radiographic changes in one of the original five patients. They confirmed their impressions of the radiographic findings by conducting animal experiments. 'Pathologic examination, when marginal indentation or 'thumbprinting' was present, revealed two possible explanations: (1) submucosal hemorrhage and (2) inflammatory areas in pericolic fat.'[1] Recognizing these 'pseudotumors' as a sign of vascular disease is important. The vascular occlusion may only be temporary and the patient's symptoms may resolve without surgical intervention.

Most historians agree that the Glasgow physician Henry Faulds' 'letter published in *Nature* [1880] represents the first writing describing fingerprints and advocating their use for the detection of criminals'[3] (Figure 2). It was Purkinje who described the nine patterns of fingerprints that make each set unique. Many earlier descriptions of finger ridges and their imprints are known from Neolithic caves discovered in first century Rome and sixth century China.

References
1. Boley, S.J., Schwartz, S., Lash, J. and Sternhill, V. (1963). Reversible vascular occlusion of the colon. *Surg. Gynecol. Obstet.*, 116, 53–60

2. Schwartz, S., Boley, S., Lash, J. and Sternhill, V. (1963). Roentgenologic aspects of reversible vascular occlusion of the colon and its relationship to ulcerative colitis. *Radiology*, 80, 625–35

3. Moenssens, A.A. (1971). The history of fingerprinting. In *Fingerprint Techniques*, pp. 1–9. (Philadelphia: Chilton Book Co.)

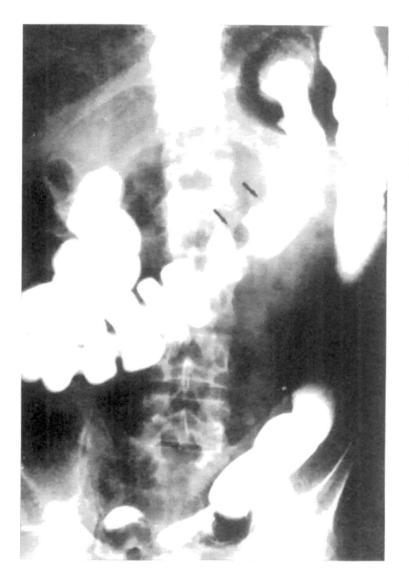

Figure 1. 'Pseudotumors ('thumbprinting') are present along the superior aspect of the transverse colon.' Reprinted from Boley et al.[1] Reversible vascular occlusion of the colon. *Surg. Gynecol. Obstet.*, 1963, **116**, 53–60, with permission of *Surgery, Gynecology & Obstetrics*, now known as the *Journal of the American College of Surgeons*

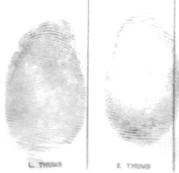

Figure 2. Identification card thumbprints

TRAM-LINE (RAILROAD TRACK) SIGN

Broncho-pulmonary aspergillosis is an infectious complication seen in some patients with chronic asthma. McCarthy and colleagues[1] (Brompton Hospital, London) related the radiographic findings of this condition in a review of 111 cases. Among the many signs they described in this article were tram-line shadows, parallel-line shadows, band-like (toothpaste) shadows and the gloved-finger shadow. Tram-line (or railroad-track) shadows were described as 'Two parallel hair-line shadows extending out from the hilum in the direction of the bronchi, the width of the transradiant zone between the lines being that of a normal bronchus'[1] (Figure 1). Parallel- line shadows were 'similar in site and direction to tram-line shadows, but the width of the trans-radiant zone between the lines is wider than that seen in a normal bronchus and, if a bronchogram is done, this bronchus will be seen to be dilated.'[1] Secretions in dilated bronchi caused toothpaste or gloved-finger shadows, thus, 'A shadow some 2–3 cm long and 5–8 mm wide is aptly described as a band-like or a toothpaste shadow ... A band-like shadow with an expanded rounded distal end can be described as a gloved-finger shadow.'[1] Such shadows are not specific for broncho-pulmonary aspergillosis. They can be seen in asthmatic patients without aspergillosis and in patients who have cystic fibrosis.

'Railways [tramways] as we know them began with ... the Industrial Revolution, in the first mines. There are illustrations in various mining textbooks from 1530 onwards showing railways or tramways, the earliest in Germany'[2] (Figure 2).

References

1. McCarthy, D.S., Simon, G. and Hargreave, F.E. (1970). The radiological appearances in allergic broncho-pulmonary aspergillosis. *Clin. Radiol.*, 21, 366–75

2. Snell, J.B. (1964). *Early Railways*, pp. 7–8. (New York: G.P. Putnam's Sons)

3. Wilson, F.E. (1961). *The British Tram*. (London: Percival Marshall and Co. Ltd)

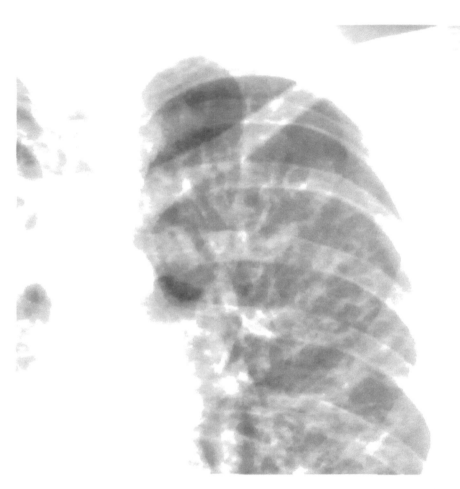

Figure 1. 'Tram-line shadows. The distance between the lines is appropriate to that of a normal bronchus at the same level.'[1] Case courtesy of Dr C. White, University of Maryland

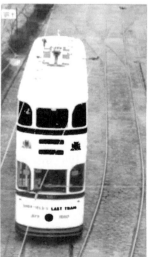

Figure 2. Sheffield tram and tracks. Photo courtesy of S. J. Gallimore, Derby, UK

TURRET EXOSTOSIS

Turret exostosis was described in 1966 by H. Andrew Wissinger, Edward McClain and Joseph Boyes[1]. They reported their findings in ten patients in the *Journal of Bone and Joint Surgery*. 'Following relatively trivial injuries to the dorsum of the proximal and middle phalanges of the fingers, a smooth, dome-shaped, extracortical collection of subperiosteal bone may develop beneath the extensor apparatus. Because of its shape and composition we have chosen to call this lesion turret exostosis'[1] (Figure 1). These exostoses usually develop several weeks to months after a lacerating injury. Wissinger said that it reminded Joseph Boyes of the gun turret on top of a World War II B-17 bomber (personal communication) (Figure 2).

The United States Army Air Corps began the development of long range (> 5000 miles) bombers in 1933. Boeing (Seattle, Washington) was awarded the development contract and the B-17's predecessor, the 299, made its debut in July 1935. 'Legend has it that one Seattle newspaperman, on seeing the plane for the first time exclaimed, 'Why it's a flying fortress!' given its size and five gun emplacements with Browning .50-caliber machine guns.' The combat debut of the Flying Fortress was in May 1941 during the Battle of Britain. Twenty B-17Cs were sold to the British under the Lend-Lease Bill signed in March 1941[2]. The B-17's successor, the B-29 Superfortress, appeared before the end of the war and is famous (or infamous) for dropping the first atomic bombs on 6 August 1945 over Hiroshima and on 9 August 1945 over Nagasaki, Japan.

References
1. Wissinger, H.A., McClain, E.J. and Boyes, J.H. (1966). Turret exostosis. *J. Bone Joint Surg.*, 48A, 105–10

2. Jablonski, E. (1965). *Flying Fortress*, pp. 3–28. (New York: Doubleday and Co. Inc.)

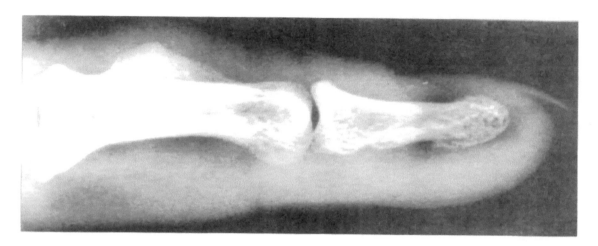

Figure 1. 'Roentgenogram made six months after injury. The turret exostosis is mature.' Reprinted from Wissinger *et al.*[1] Turret exostosis. *J. Bone Joint Surg.*, 1966, **48A**, 105–110, with permission of the editor

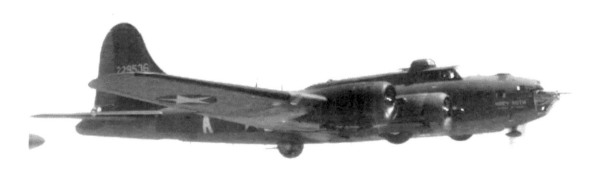

Figure 2. B-17 with top gun turret visible. Courtesy of the National Air and Space Museum, Smithsonian Institution, Washington, DC

WATERFALL HILUM

Larry Elliott and Gerold Schiebler[1] (then at University of Florida) in their book, *The X-ray Diagnosis of Congenital Heart Disease in Infants, Children, and Adults,* ascribe this distinct sign of pulmonary shunt vascularity (Figure 1) to Kent Ellis. Shunt vascularity is another one of the key findings to look for when evaluating the chest radiograph in cases of congenital heart disease (see Egg shaped heart, Mogul shadow and Shmoo shaped heart). In the book, Elliott reported that the most common congenital heart condition prone to show the 'waterfall right hilum' sign is transposition of the great vessels with a single ventricle.[1] 'The other complex lesions [transposition, tricuspid atresia, truncus arteriosus], most notably complete transposition with a large [ventricular septal defect] VSD, may uncommonly show the same finding ... the so-called 'waterfall right hilum' sign. It is produced by the combination of torrential and increased pulmonary flow plus an elevation of the right pulmonary artery (RPA) itself. The elevation of the RPA is caused by massive dilatation of the pulmonary trunk, which, in turn, causes an uplifting of the RPA.'[1]

A waterfall is an 'area where flowing river water drops abruptly and nearly vertically [much like the descending right pulmonary artery] (Figure 2). The highest waterfall in the world is the Angel Fall in Venezuela (807 m [2,650 ft]).'[2] Niagara Falls, on the United States/Canadian border, has one of the largest flow volumes of any waterfall in the world. It averages about 195 000 cubic feet per second.

References

1. Elliott, L.P. and Schiebler, G.L. (1979). *The X-ray Diagnosis of Congenital Heart Disease in Infants, Children, and Adults.* 2nd edn, pp. 379–83. (Springfield, IL: Charles C. Thomas)

2. Waterfall. In *The New Encyclopaedia Britannica,* 1990, 15th edn, Vol. 12, p. 521. (Chicago: Encyclopaedia Britannica Inc.)

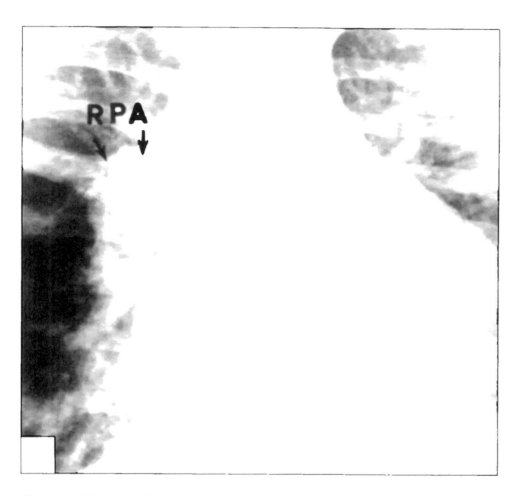

Figure 1. 'Cyanosis and shunt with elevated right pulmonary artery (RPA) (waterfall hilum).' Reprinted from *The X-ray Diagnosis of Congenital Heart Disease in Infants, Children and Adults* by Elliot and Schiebler (1979)[1], with permission. Courtesy of Charles C. Thomas, Publisher, Springfield, Il

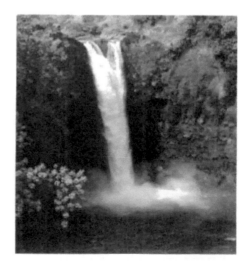

Figure 2. Rainbow Falls (near Hilo, Hawaii)

WINE GOBLET (WINE GLASS) SIGN

Luis Surraco[1] (Montevideo, Uruguay) coined the 'goblet sign' term to describe the pyelographic appearance of some renal hydatid cysts (Figure 1). He reported 29 cases, the largest group in the medical literature at the time (1939). '[T]he cyst never opens directly into the pelvis of the kidney without having its base always resting *upon the end of a primary calyx* through a solitary and small hole of communication. As a result of this, we note a special aspect of the cyst: the aspect which will give rise to the pyelographic indication which I have called the 'goblet sign'. This sign consists in a large oval cavity represented by the pericystium, with one base of support upon the extremity of the primary calyx, and with one support represented by this primary calyx.'[1]

The term was later applied[2] to the somewhat similar 'cup-shaped deformity' in the ureter caused by ureteral tumors[3] (Figure 2). The unique feature seen during excretory urography with this sign is widening of the ureter just below the tumoral filling defect. This contrasts with ureteral narrowing typically seen at the level of a ureteral calculus. Recognition of this radiographic sign is important since 'there [were] no recognized signs and symptoms characteristic of ureteral tumor'[3] before this and the clinical symptoms (pain) and signs (hematuria) may be the same with either tumor or stone.

'Wine is the fermented juice of the grape. Of the grape genus *Vitis*, one species, *V. vinifera*, is used almost exclusively'[4] for the production of wine. Wines, and the vessels (glasses, goblets) used to consume them, have a long history. 'Wine had a history by the time the Old Testament was written; in Genesis 9:20 it is ascribed to Noah.'[5] '*Vitis vinifera* was being cultivated in the Middle East by 4000 BC, and probably earlier.'[4] (Figure 3 shows a wine glass.)

References

1. Surraco, L.A. (1939). Renal hydatidosis. *Am. J. Surg.*, 44, 581–6

2. Wood, L.G. and Howe, G.E. (1958). Primary tumors of the ureter: case reports. *J. Urol.*, 79, 418–30

3. Hamm, F.C. and Lavalle, L.L. (1949). Tumors of the ureter. *J. Urol.*, 61, 493–505

4 Beverage production. In *The New Encyclopaedia Britannica*, 1990, 15th edn, Vol. 14, pp. 734–54. (Chicago: Encyclopaedia Britannica Inc.)

5. Wine. In *The New Encyclopaedia Britannica*, 1990, 15th edn, Vol. 12, p. 702. (Chicago: Encyclopaedia Britannica Inc.)

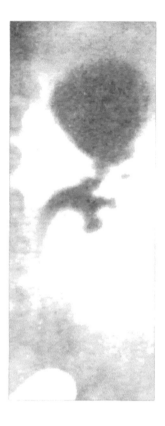

Figure 1. 'Open hydatid cyst, showing the goblet sign.' Reprinted from Surraco[1]. Renal hydaticlosis. *Am. J. Surg.*, **44,** 581–6, with permission from *American Journal of Surgery*

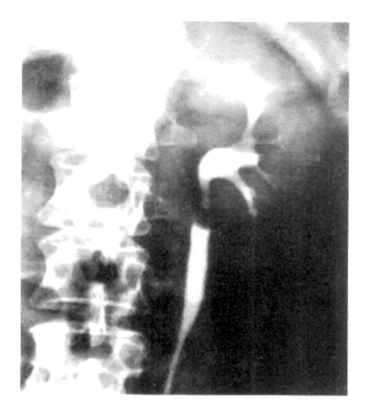

Figure 2. Ureter with goblet deformity due to ureteral tumor. Reprinted from Wood and Howe[2]. Primary tumors of the ureter. *J. Urol.,* 1958, **79,** 418–430, with permission of Williams & Wilkins

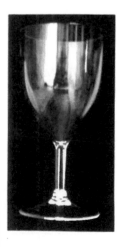

Figure 3. A wine glass or goblet

PHOTOGRAPHY CREDITS

Apple core (napkin ring) lesion: Figure 2 — original by M.E.M.*

Bamboo spine: Figure 1 — original by D.C.†; Figure 2 — original by M.E.M.

Beak (claw) sign: Figure 2 — original by M.E.M.

Beaten silver (beaten brass) pattern: Figure 2 — original by M.E.M.

Blade of grass (flame or 'V') sign: Figure 2 — original by D.C.; Figure 3 — original by M.E.M.

Boot-shaped heart (coeur en sabot): Figure 2 — original D.C.

Butterfly and bat's wing shadow: Figure 3 — original by M.E.M.

Button sequestrum: Figure 2 — original by M.E.M.

Camalote (waterlily) sign: Figure 2 — original by M.E.M.

Carpenter's level sign: Figure 1 — supplied by the original authors; Figure 2 — original by M.E.M.

Celery-stick (celery stalk) metaphysis: Figure 2 — original by M.E.M.

Cloverleaf skull: Figure 1 — original by D.C.; Figure 2 — original by M.E.M.

Cobblestone pattern: Figure 1— original by D.C.

Codfish (fish) vertebra: Figure 2 — original by D.C.

Coffee bean sign: Figure 2 — original by M.E.M.

Coin lesion: Figure 1 — original D.C.; Figure 2 — original by M.E.M.

Cookie bite (cookie cutter) lesions: Figure 2 — original by M.E.M.

Corduroy (cloth) vertebra: Figure 1 — original by D.C.; Figure 2 — original by M.E.M.

Cotton wool sign: Figure 2 — original by M.E.M.

Crescent sign: Figure 2 — supplied by Lick Observatory

Cupid's bow vertebra: Figure 2 — original by D.C.

Delta (empty triangle) sign: Figure 2 — original by D.C.

Doughnut sign: Figure 2 — original by D.C.; Figure 3 — original by M.E.M.

Dripping candlewax sign: Figure 1 — original by D.C.; Figure 2 – original by M.E.M.

Egg shaped (egg-on-a-string) heart: Figure 2 — original by M.E.M.

Egg-shell calcifications: Figure 2 — original by D.C.; Figure 3 — original by M.E.M.

Erlenmeyer flask deformity: Figure 2 — original by M.E.M.

Football sign: Figure 2 — original by M.E.M.

Greenstick fracture: Figure 1 — original by D.C.; Figure 2 — original by M.E.M.

Ground glass pattern: Figures 2 and 3 — originals by D.C.

Gull wings and mouse ears: Figure 1 — original by D.C.

Hair-on-end pattern: Figure 2 — original by M.E.M.

Hitch-hiker's thumb: Figure 2 — original by M.E.M.

Honda ('H') sign: Figure 2 — original by M.E.M.

Honeycomb lung: Figures 1 and 2 — originals by D.C.

Horseshoe kidney: Figure 2 — original by D.C.; Figure 3 — original by M.E.M.

Iceberg (tip of the iceberg) sign: Figure 2 — supplied by the US Coast Guard

Ivory vertebra: Figures 2A and 2B — originals by D.C.

---

*M.E.M. is Michael E. Mulligan.
† D.C. is David Crandall

Lead (gas) pipe sign: Figure 2 — original by M.E.M.

Lemon and banana signs: Figures 4 and 5 — originals by M.E.M.

Leontiasis ossea: Figure 1 — original by D.C.; Figure 3 — original by M.EM.

Lincoln log (H-shaped) vertebra: Figure 2 — original by D.C.

Linguine (free-floating loose thread) sign: Figure 2 — original by M.E.M.

Mallet (baseball) finger: Figure 1 — original by D.C.

Mercedes-Benz (Mercedes star) sign: Figures 2 and 3 — originals by M.E.M.

Miliary pattern: Figures 1 and 2 — originals by D.C.

Napoleon hat (bow) sign: Figure 1 — original by D.C.

Onion skin sign: Figure 2 — original by M.E.M.

Parchment heart: Figure 3 — original by M.E.M.

Phrygian cap gallbladder: Figure 1 — original by D.C.

Picket fence and stack of coins signs: Figures 3 and 4 — originals by M.E.M.

Picture frame sign: Figure 2 and 3 originals by D.C.

Playboy bunny: Figure 2 — supplied by Playboy Enterprises Inc. (PEI)

Porcelain gallbladder: Figure 1 — original by D.C.; Figure 2 — original by M.E.M.

Pruned tree and leafless tree signs: Figure 2 — original M.E.M.

Ribbon (twisted ribbon) ribs: Figure 2 — original by M.E.M.

'S' (Golden's) sign: Figure 2 — original by M.E.M.

Saber-sheath trachea: Figure 2 — original by M.E.M.

Sabre shin: Figure 1 — original by D.C.; Figure — 2 original by M.E.M.

Sail and spinnaker sail signs: Figure 2 — supplied by the US Navy

Sausage (cocktail sausage) digit: Figure 1 — original by D.C.; Figure 2 — original by M.E.M.

Scottie dog: Figure 2 — original by D.C.

Shepherd's crook: Figure 1 — original by M.E.M.

Silhouette sign: Figure 2 — original by M.E.M.

Silver forks: Figure 1 and 2 — originals by D.C.

Snowman (figure-8) sign: Figure 2 — original by M.E.M.

Spinning top (arrowhead) urethra: Figure 2 — original by M.E.M.

Staghorn calculi: Figure 2 — original by M.E.M.

String sign: Figure 2 — original by M.E.M.

Tear-drop sign: Figure 2 — original by M.E.M.

Telephone receiver femur: Figure 2 — original by M.E.M.

Terry-Thomas and signet rings sign: Figure 4 — original by M.E.M.

Thumbprinting sign: Figure 2 — original by M.E.M.

Tram-line (railroad track) sign: Figure 1 — original by D.C.; Figure 2 — original by S.J. Gallimore

Waterfall hilum: Figure 2 — original by M.E.M.

Wine goblet (wine glass) sign: Figure 3 — original by M.E.M.

SUBJECT INDEX

NAME INDEX

T - #0524 - 071024 - C208 - 246/189/10 - PB - 9780367401153 - Gloss Lamination